Biology
for Engineers

Biology
for Engineers

for **Students of BTech and BE Courses**

Based on Syllabus Prescribed by AICTE for
Engineering and Technology Course Curriculum, 2018

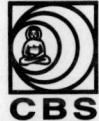

Rajiv Singal MBBS MS
Vice Chairman
RPIIT Technical and Medical Campus, Karnal (Haryana)

Gaurav Agarwal M Pharm (BITS-Pilani) PhD
Dean, Faculty of Pharmacy
RPIIT, Karnal (Haryana)

Ritu Bir MSc MPhil
Assistant Professor
Delhi College of Technology and Management
Palwal (Haryana)

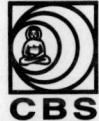

CBS

CBS Publishers & Distributors Pvt Ltd

New Delhi • Bengaluru • Chennai • Kochi • Kolkata • Lucknow • Mumbai
Hyderabad • Jharkhand • Nagpur • Patna • Pune • Uttarakhand

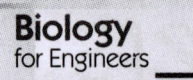

Biology
for Engineers ___

ISBN: 978-93-88902-78-6

Copyright © Authors and Publisher

First Edition: 2019

Reprint: 2020², 2022, 2024

Published by Satish Kumar Jain and Produced by Varun Jain for

CBS Publishers & Distributors Pvt Ltd

4819/XI Prahlad Street, 24 Ansari Road, Daryaganj, New Delhi 110 002, India.   4819/XI Prahlad Street, 24 Ansari Road, Daryaganj, New Delhi 110 002, India.

Ph: 23289259, 23266861

Website: www.cbspd.com
e-mail: delhi@cbspd.com

Corporate Office: 204 FIE, Industrial Area, Patparganj, Delhi 110 092

Ph: 011-4934 4934   Fax: 011-4934 4935

e-mail: publishing@cbspd.com;
publicity@cbspd.com

Branches

- **Bengaluru:** Seema House 2975, 17th Cross, K.R. Road, Banasankari 2nd Stage, Bengaluru 560 070, Karnataka
  Ph: +91-80-26771678/79   Fax: +91-80-26771680   e-mail: bangalore@cbspd.com
- **Chennai:** 7, Subbaraya Street, Shenoy Nagar, Chennai 600 030, Tamil Nadu, India
  Ph: +91-44-26680620/26681266   Fax: +91-44-42032115   e-mail: chennai@cbspd.com
- **Kochi:** 42/1325, 1326, Power House Road, Opp KSEB, Power House, Ernakulam 682 018, Kochi, Kerala, India
  Ph: +91-484-4059061-65, 67   Fax: +91-484-4059065   e-mail: kochi@cbspd.com
- **Kolkata:** 147, Hind Ceramics Compound, 1st Floor, Nilgunj Road, Belghoria, Kolkata-700056, West Bengal, India
  Ph: +033-25633055, 033-25633056   e-mail: kolkata@cbspd.com
- **Lucknow:** Basement, Khushnuma Complex, 7 Meerabai Marg (Behind Jawahar Bhawan), Lucknow-226001, UP, India
  Ph: +91-522-4000032   e-mail: tiwari.lucknow@cbspd.com
- **Mumbai:** PWD Shed, Gala no 25/26, Ramchandra Bhatt Marg, Next to JJ Hospital Gate no. 2, Opp. Union Bank of India Noorbaug, Mumbai-400009, Maharashtra, India
  Ph: 022-66661880/89   e-mail: mumbai@cbspd.com

Representatives

- **Hyderabad**   0-9885175004
- **Patna**   0-9334159340
- **Jharkhand**   0-9811541605
- **Pune**   0-9664372571
- **Nagpur**   0-8692091830
- **Uttarakhand**   0-9716462459

Printed at Glorious Printer, Dilshad Garden, Delhi, India

to
_____

my loving kids
Mansi and **Saloni**

Foreword

It gives me a great pleasure to comment on the book entitled *Biology for Engineers* by Dr Rajiv Singal, Dr Gaurav Agarwal and Mrs Ritu Bir. This book is a thoughtful compilation of many topics of biology. It has taken rapid strides over the last few decades in understanding various concepts related to topics of biology. The efforts have been mainly taken to focus on the primary aspects of biology for students undergoing degree and diploma courses of various degree/diploma awarding bodies. Although the efforts have been mainly concentrated on the entry-level students, the book covers a wide range of areas in brief and contains a comprehensive description. I am confident that it will be an appropriate effort to prove its utility for engineering students. Biology, being an interdisciplinary subject today, is covering a wide range of interest both among the students and teaching communities. The basic text in simple language not only deals with the basic concepts but also emphasizes technical and practical aspects of the subject.

The main objective of the book is to explain the fundamentals of biology in the simplest possible language easy to understand by all the students and the authors have been successful in their objectives. I am glad to note that the present textbook keeps the balance between the basics essential and advance areas of knowledge in biology.

Authors should be congratulated for the tremendous efforts they have taken in compiling this useful work for the budding technocrats. I am pleased to introduce the book for engineering students.

Prof (Dr) Pardeep
Pro Vice-Chancellor
Galgotias University
Greater Noida, UP

Preface

This book *Biology for Engineers* is designed specifically for BTech third semester students as per course curriculum, 2018 prescribed by AICTE.

This book, although designated for entry-level students, covers wide areas. It contains a comprehensive description, an overview of existing knowledge of biology and making it appropriate for introductory and institutional purposes.

Being an interdisciplinary subject, it is today covering a wide range of interest both among the students and teaching communities. Taking this increasing interest into account, this book gives a comprehensive introduction to the subject. The text not only deals with the basic concepts but also emphasizes technical and practical aspects of the subject. The book is primarily intended as text for engineering students.

The book contains numerous specimens, vivid illustrations, tables, diagrams and flow diagrams to present the ideas. The distinguishing feature is ample question bank at the end of each chapter. The structure and the content of the book have changed to reflect modern thinking and current university curricula throughout the world. In spite of great care there might be some mistakes and deficiencies and we will be grateful to the readers for giving suggestions to improve upon ourself. So go through the content and do mail at *gbitsian@rediffmail.com*.

Rajiv Singal
Gaurav Agarwal
Ritu Bir

Acknowledgements

It is a moment of a great pleasure and immense satisfaction for us to express deep gratitude and gratefulness to Shri RP Singal, Chairman, RP Educational Trust, for inspiring us to bring out this book.

Our special thanks to Er Bharat Singal and Anuj Singal, Secretary, RP Educational Trust, for their all time support and encouragement.

We express our gratefulness to Shri YN Arjuna, Senior Vice President–Publishing, Editorial and Publicity, and special thanks to Shri Satish K Jain, CMD, CBS Publishers & Distributors for their sincere efforts.

Last but not the least, we express our love to our family and friends for their all time inspiration and dedication. They were always a constant source of motivation in bringing out this book!

To our numerous students, whom we cannot possibly name individually, we thank for their class interactions which have been the guiding spirit in selection of the subject matter and its logical arrangement.

Rajiv Singal
Gaurav Agarwal

I would like to acknowledge the large heartedness of my family and colleagues. My family was supportive from the beginning and encouraged me to write this book. I would like to pay my gratitude to my parents for their blessings. I would like to acknowledge the motivation of my loving husband Dr P Kumar who encouraged me throughout writing this book. My children, Paarth and Naman, deserve a special hug for the patience and concern shown towards me to complete this book.

This book is dedicated to all the students to whom I have taught at DCTM, Palwal, Haryana. I hope students will appreciate this book.

At last I would like to thank the Almighty.

Ritu Bir

Contents

Chapter 1

Introduction to Biology

SYNOPSIS

This chapter will cover the following topics

1. Importance of biology as an integral part of other field of Science like Mathematics, Physics and Chemistry.
2. Study the fundamental differences between science and engineering by comparison between eye and camera, bird flying and aircraft.
3. Biology as an independent scientific discipline.
4. Need to study biology.
5. Discuss how biological observations of 18th century that lead to major discoveries.
6. Examples from Brownian motion and the origin of thermodynamics, observation of Robert Brown and Julius Mayor.

INTRODUCTION OF SCIENCE

The word science implies the knowledge, understanding and implementation of phenomenon occurring in the universe relevant to human beings. It is learned through experiments and observation in a particular area or branch of scientific study such as biology, physics, chemistry or mathematics or any other branch of the natural or physical science.

Integration of Branches of Science

Science is broadly studied in four major branches, i.e. **Biology, Physics, Chemistry** and **Mathematics**. These branches are further divided into various subjects of study. Although no perfect definition of these branches can be given but to understand, we can say that biology is the science of living organism, chemistry is the study of matter, physics is the study of force and energy and mathematics is a study of derivations and calculations.

All these branches of science are not a separate entity in itself; rather they are integrated through various functions and phenomenon. For example, in biology the basic unit of life is cell and cell itself contains many types of chemical and enzymes to produce energy and other functions and the various functions like growth, movement involve mathematical calculations. Now, we understand that there is interlining of various branches of science.

To draw out comparison between biology and engineering we will discuss the following examples.

Eye and Camera

In Fig. 1.1 and Tables 1.1 and 1.2 structure of camera and human eye along with the similarities and difference is explained.

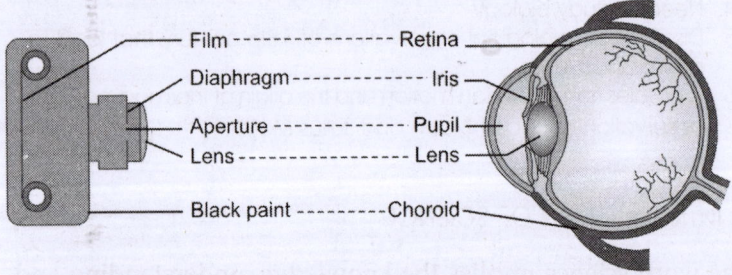

Fig. 1.1: Comparison between camera and human eye

Bird and Aircraft

Both birds and planes are capable of flying and the science has shown that a principle behind this ability of flying in both cases is same but the mechanism is different.

The basic principle of flying is based on Bernoulli's principle

The particles in air are always moving. Air like a fluid will always move from a high pressure area to a low pressure. He found that fast moving air has lower pressure and slow moving

Table 1.1 Similarities between camera and human eye

Part of the camera	Corresponding part of an eye	Function
Aperture	Pupil	Light enters the eye through the pupil/aperture
Diaphragm	Iris	The iris/diaphragm regulates the amount of light entering the eye/camera.
Lens	Lens	Focus light and image on the retina in eye and film in camera
Film	Retina	The part on which images are formed
Black paint	Choroid	The dark-colored melanin pigment in the choroid and black paint in camera absorbs light and limits reflections within the eye that could degrade vision

Table 1.2 Differences between camera and human eye

Camera	Human eye
Focal length of lens is fixed	Focal length of the lens can be changed
Photographic film retains the image permanently	Retina retains the impression of an image for only $1/16^{th}$ second
A photograph has to be changed for getting next image	Same retina can be used for viewing unlimited images
Image is formed on photographic film and processing can be done through computer	Image is formed on retina which is further processed in brain

air has higher pressure. It is this Bernoulli's principle that helped us how birds and airplanes can fly.

When air rushes past the wing of a plane, it flows above and below the wing. The top part of the wing is rounded and the bottom is fairly straight. Therefore, air rushing over the top of the wing has to travel a greater distance to the back of the wing compared to the bottom (Fig. 1.2).

As a result, the air on the top of the wing has to travel faster to keep up with the air underneath. This creates a low pressure area on the top of the wing and high pressure area on the bottom. The difference of pressures on the surfaces of the wing creates **lift** (the upward force that keeps planes and birds aloft.)

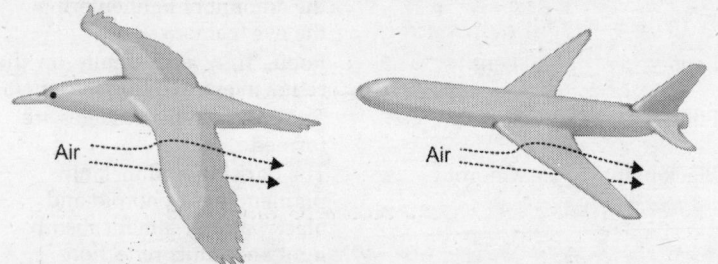

Fig. 1.2: Forces that act on birds during flight

1. **Lift:** The force that pushes upward, created by the movement of air over and under the wings.
2. **Drag:** The force of the air pressing against the bird and slowing them down.
3. **Thrust:** The force that moves the bird forward, caused when a bird flaps its wings.
4. **Propulsion:** It means to push forward or drive an object forward. A propulsion system is a machine that produces thrust.

   Newton's Third Law: For every action there is an equal and opposite reaction. Thrust often comes from muscles or engines.

Characteristics of Birds

Important things that birds have that help them keep their weight low are:

1. **Feathers**—are light, flexible, used for protection and also to keep the bird warm.
2. **Hollow bones**—are very light
3. Strong muscles.

A comparison between flying of aeroplane and flying of birds is shown in Table 1.3.

Table 1.3 Comparison between flying of aeroplanes and birds

Function	Part of the aeroplane	Part of the bird
Lift	Propellers/airfoil	Muscles
Drag	Streamlined shape	Light weight skeleton and streamlined shape
Thrust	Movement of aeroplanes and wings by engine	Flapping of wings
Control	Wings	Tail and wings
Propulsion	Engine	Muscles

Biology as an independent scientific discipline

Biology is one of the interesting subjects of science as it is directly related to our day-to-day life. The main difference between biology and other subjects of science that biology is not limited to laboratory only. It goes beyond labs into forest, oceans, hills, etc., i.e. it brings us closer to the nature. Following are the few examples of interesting facts which helps us developing interest in biology as subject:

1. Did you ever wonder why the colour of our blood is red? The answer is the iron present in our blood forms a ring of atoms called porphyrin, the shape of this structure produces the red colour.

2. Human bone is an excellent example of a perfect architecture. The femur that supports the weight of our body during walking is more powerful when compared to a solid concrete of the same weight.

3. What's the largest organ of the human body? Quite surprising, but the answer is your skin.

4. The relation between your thumb and your nose is—the length of your thumb is equal to the length of your nose.

5. Every nucleus in the human body has DNA of 6 feet long.

6. Magnetoreception is a type of magnetic compass present in some migratory birds that help them navigate using the Earth's magnetic field.

7. Curious to know how **dolphins** sleep? Then, here you go, dolphins sleep half awake. They keep one eye open while they consciously breathe and float on the water surface.

8. The **ostrich egg** is the biggest in the world. It equals to the volume of as much as 30 chicken eggs.

9. The life of an eyelash is no more than 5 months.

10. What is the largest flower in the world? **Rafflesia Arnoldii**. It can grow as big as an umbrella.

11. Now, that you know about the world's largest flower, you must also know about the world's smallest flowering plant, **Wolffia**. One full bouquet of its flowers fits on the head of a push pin.

12. Armadillos spend about 80% of their life asleep! Did you know?

13. How do ants eat? Want to know? Ants cannot chew their food, they move their jaws sideways like scissors to extract the juices from the food.

14. In seahorses, the male gives birth to a young one.

15. Do you know human's nose and ears? They do not stop growing

Need to Study Biology

Biology is an interesting subject that has been intriguing scientific minds for several centuries. Biology has an endless array of species (at least as of now because there are an estimated 8.7 million species on earth out of which only 1.9 million species have been discovered, so there is a long way to go). Every creation which is a part of nature is so adorable and unique in its own way.

Biology exists every second—when we inhale and exhale each time, respiration is taking place within our bodies, each cell receives oxygenated blood and releases carbon dioxide and other excretory wastes.

Let aside other species, we haven't yet understood our own bodies completely. How is it that our hearts work so tirelessly throughout our life span, how is it that we are able to interpret even minute emotions and gestures without even under-standing the mechanism behind it? How is it that each one of us is able to perceive things differently? What exactly is consciousness? The list of questions seeking their answers is endless!

Ecology, for example, studies the relationship between animals, plants, and the environment, helping us understand how the things humans and other animals do can hurt or help Nature.

Immunology studies our immune system and how it reacts to all sorts of different threats.

Pathology diagnoses diseases and what causes them, as well as what they do to the body. Virology does the same for the many different viruses that may cause harm to us.

The study of biology has helped humans to understand the similarities between all forms of life. For example, the genetic code that helps to construct all living organisms is very similar in all life forms. The genetic material is stored in the form of DNA for all plants, animals, bacteria and fungi. By studying the DNA of all these different life forms, biologists have determined that all living creatures are related to each other.

Biology has also helped doctors learn how to keep people healthy and fight off disease. Biologists have learned that things called pathogens, which are themselves other living entities, cause diseases. By understanding how these dangerous organisms work, scientists can fight them off. Because of biology, many people have lived long lives as they have been able to avoid diseases.

Biology also studies the origin of diseases and plagues, such as infections, pathologies of animals and damage to plants and trees. Biology encompasses the study of the functions of living beings, enhancement of useful species, factors that cause illnesses, discovery and production of medicines and sustainable use of natural resources. Through biotechnology, biologists find efficient ways to produce food and other supplies for people. They investigate the processes involved in producing various nutritional substances.

Observations of 18th Century

Aristotle was one of these first biologists and pursued finding the core of human intelligence, which he concluded to be the heart. Aristotle was a Greek philosopher who studied human anatomy and marine science.

1. The work of many naturalist explorers like Humboldt (1769–1859), Bonpland (1773–1858) greatly increased European appreciation of the enormous extent of the diversity and geographical variation of plants, animals, and fungi. During the eighteenth century great labors were dedicated to the collection, preservation, and cataloging of flora and fauna.

2. The need to organize the resultant wealth of information motivated the work of Carl Linnaeus (1707–1778), who laid the foundations for the modern system of binomial nomenclature.

3. The chemical discoveries of Lavoisier (1743–1794) were instrumental in the development of physiology and biophysics in the following century.

4. Edward Jenner (1749 –1823) was an English physician and scientist who was the pioneer of smallpox vaccine, the world's first vaccine. The terms "vaccine" and "vaccination" are derived from Variolae vaccinae (smallpox of the cow), the term devised by Jenner to denote cowpox Jenner is often called "the father of immunology", and his work is said to have "saved more lives than the work of any other human".

5. Hanaoka Seishû (1760–1835) was a Japanese surgeon. Hanaoka is said to have been the first to perform surgery using general anesthesia.

Brownian motion and the origin of thermodynamics

During microscopic research performed in 1827, Brown made his biggest discovery. While observing the sexual organs of plants under the microscope, the scientist found that pollen grains seemed to be darting around in a random manner. Curious, Brown studied other substances under the microscope in search of the same movement. He discovered that if particles were of a certain size (or smaller), that the movement continued to occur. Brown observed the same movement in glass and rock particles, and theorized that the movement was not limited to living matter. The botanist concluded that the movement was caused by some phenomenon of physics and named the phenomenon "Brownian motion." In 1905, Albert Einstein suggested that Brownian motion was the result of the particles colliding with molecules. Nobel Prize winner, Jean Perrin, proved that Einstein's thesis of Brownian motion was correct. Brown's discovery provided the first evidence that proved the existence of atoms. The phenomenon of Brownian motion also led scientists to quantify Avagadro's number—a physical constant for describing random motion.

Brownian motion is the continuous random **movement** of small particles suspended in a fluid, which arise from collisions with the fluid molecules. **Examples of Brownian motion are:**

1. The motion of pollen grains on still water
2. Movement of dust motes in a room (although largely affected by air currents)
3. Diffusion of pollutants in air
4. Diffusion of calcium through bones
5. Movement of "holes" of electrical charge in semiconductors

Importance of Brownian Motion

The initial importance of defining and describing Brownian motion was that it supported the modern atomic theory. Today, the mathematical models that describe Brownian motion are used in mathematics, economics, engineering, physics, biology, chemistry, and a host of other disciplines.

Overview: Robert Mayer

In thermodynamics, **Julius Robert Mayer** (1814–1878) was a German physician and physicist notable for making one of the first statements of the conservation of energy and the mechanical equivalent of heat, namely that "motion is converted into heat" (1841), in contrast to the caloric theory, and for making a crude calculation of the latter.

Observation of Robert Mayer that led to the Concept of Thermodynamics

In 1840, Mayer was travelling in a ship destined for a roundtrip to Java. On this voyage two curiosities came to interest him.

First, he was told by the navigator that during a storm the ocean water becomes warmer. This meant, to Mayer, that the agitation, motion, or mechanical action of the waves had been converted into heat. A second note, observed by Mayer, was that during his blood letting procedures he noticed that the venous blood, which is normally a blue colored type of blood being carried in vessels from the capillaries towards the heart, was redder in color than expected.

Laws of Thermodynamics

1. The first law of thermodynamics is an extension of the law of conservation of energy
2. The second law can also be stated that heat flows sponta-neously from a hot object to a cold object (spontaneously means without the assistance of external work)

   Automobile engines, refrigerators, and air conditioners all work on the principles laid out by the second law of Thermo-dynamics. Ever wonder why you can't cool your kitchen in the hot summer by leaving the refrigerator door open? Feel the air coming off the back—you heat the air outside to cool the air inside.

   The Zeroth Law states that if A is in thermal equilibrium with B, and B is in equilibrium with object C, then C is also in thermal equilibrium with A.

Examples of the First and Second Law of Thermodynamics

Melting Ice Cube

Every day, ice needs to be maintained at a temperature below the freezing point of water to remain solid. On hot summer days, however, people often take out a tray of ice to cool bever-ages. In the process, they witness the first and second laws of thermodynamics. For example, someone might put an ice cube into a glass of warm lemonade and then forget to drink the beverage. An hour or two later, they will notice that the ice has melted but the temperature of the lemonade has cooled. This is because the total amount of heat in the system has remained the same, but has just gravitated towards equilibrium, where both the former ice cube (now water) and the lemonade are the same temperature. This is, of course, not a completely closed system. The lemonade will eventually become warm again, as heat from the environment is transferred to the glass and its contents.

Sweating in a Crowded Room

The human body obeys the laws of thermodynamics. Consider the experience of being in a small crowded room with lots of other people. In all likelihood, you'll start to feel very warm and will start sweating. This is the process your body uses to cool itself off. Heat from your body is transferred to the sweat. As the sweat absorbs more and more heat, it evaporates from your body, becoming more disordered and transferring heat to the air, which heats up the air temperature of the room. Many sweating people in a crowded room, "closed system," will quickly heat things up. This is both the first and second laws of thermodynamics in action: No heat is lost; it is merely transferred.

Flipping a Light Switch

We rely on electricity to turn on our lights. Electricity is a form of energy; it is, however, a secondary source. A primary source of energy must be converted into electricity before we can flip on the lights. For example, water energy can be harnessed by building a dam to hold back the water of a large lake. If we slowly release water through a small opening in the dam, we can use the driving pressure of the water to turn a turbine. The work of the turbine can be used to generate electricity with the help of a generator. The electricity is sent to our homes via power lines. The electricity was not created out of nothing; it is the result of transforming water energy from the lake into another energy form.

KEY POINTS

- Science is broadly studied in four major branches, i.e. **Biology, Physics, Chemistry** and **Mathematics**.

- Both birds and planes are capable of flying and the science has shown that a principle behind this ability of flying in both cases is same but the mechanism is different.
- The basic principle of flying is based on Bernoulli's principle
- Newton's Third Law: For every action there is an equal and opposite reaction.
- Biology exists every second: When we inhale and exhale each time, respiration is taking place within our bodies, each cell receives oxygenated blood and releases carbon dioxide and other excretory wastes.
- Immunology studies our immune system and how it reacts to all sorts of different threats.
- Pathology diagnoses diseases and what causes them, as well as what they do to the body.
- The genetic material is stored in the form of DNA for all plants, animals, bacteria and fungi.
- Aristotle was a Greek philosopher who studied human anatomy and marine science.
- **Brownian motion** is the continuous random **movement** of small particles suspended in a fluid, which arise from collisions with the fluid molecules.
- **Laws of thermodynamics:**
  1. The first law of thermodynamics is an extension of the law of conservation of energy.
  2. The second law can also be stated that heat flows spontaneously from a hot object to a cold object (spontaneously means without the assistance of external work).

PRACTICE QUESTIONS

Very Short Answer Type Questions

1. Give one example of Brownian motion.
2. What is biology?
3. What is Brownian motion?

4. Give example of first law of thermodynamics.

5. What basic principle of flying is used by birds?

Long Answer Type Questions

1. What is the need to study for biology?

2. Give example of Brownian motion.

3. Give differences between (a) flying bird and aeroplane (b) camera and eye.

4. Which features help a bird to fly?

Classification System in Biology

This chapter will cover the following topics

1. Classification as well as morphological, biochemical or ecological parameters are highlighted. Hierarchy of life forms at phenomenological level.
2. Discuss about classification at (a) Cellularity—unicellular or multicellular, (b) Ultrastructure—prokaryotes or eukaryotes, (c) Energy and carbon utilisation—autotrophs, heterotrophs, lithotropes, (d) Ammonia excretion—amminotelic, uricotelic, ureotelic, (e) Habitat—aquatic or terrestrial, (f) Molecular taxonomy.
3. Study of Model organisms *E. coli, S. cerevisiae, D. Melanogaster, C. elegance, A. Thaliana, M. musculus.*

IMPORTANT TERMS RELATED TO CLASSIFICATION/TAXONOMY

1. Nomenclature: It is the process of giving scientific names (not vernacular or local names) to the organisms.
2. Classification: It is the process of grouping animals and plants into convenient categories on the basis of certain observable traits.
3. Identification: It is determination of correct position of an organism in the classification.
4. Taxonomy: It is the study of the process of classification.
5. Systematic: This includes the identification, nomenclature and classification of organisms based on various parameters.
6. New systematic: This covers systematic studies considering evolutionary relationship including other branches like

molecular biology, cytology, genetics, and biochemistry, etc.

HISTORY OF CLASSIFICATION

1. Hippocrates—he classified animals into various groups like insects, fishes and birds, etc.
2. Aristotle—known as father of zoology/biology. He had written Historia animalium.
3. Theophrastus—known as father of botany
4. John Ray (1686)—a British botanist.
5. Carrolus Linnaeus—a Swedish naturalist—Father of taxonomy. He coined the terms 'class' and 'systematics. Taxonomy was given by AP De Condolle. He published 'Systema Naturae, Genera Plantarum and Species Plantarum (1753)'.

ROLE OF NOMENCLATURE

1. In bionomial nomenclature each scientific name has 2 components:
   i. Generic name (Genus)
   ii. Specific name/epithet (Species)
2. The generic name begins with capital letter, whereas the specific name with small letter
3. Both the generic and specific names are separately underlined (if handwritten), or given in italic (if printed) to indicate their Latin origin.
4. The first (generic) name is usually a noun, whereas the second (species) is an adjective.
5. The scientific name of the organism is generally followed by the name (full or abbreviated) of the person/author, who first described the species. However if the species, after its first publication is transferred to any other genus, or the generic name is changed, the first author's name is given in parenthesis (brackets). If the specific name is given in the honor of a person, then this name ends in 'i' if the person is male or in 'ae' if the honor person is female.

6. Tautonym—it is a bionomial name in which the names of genus and species are the same.
7. Julian Huxley—introduced the term 'New-systematics'
8. Whittaker (1969)—introduced 5 kingdoms classification.

INTRODUCTION

The basic unit of biological classification is known as species. According to the biological concept of the species they can be defined as group of natural population of animals and plants, whose members can interbreed among themselves and reproductively isolated from other such groups. It is not applicable to fossils and asexually reproducing organisms as they cannot interbreed. So far, there are more than 1.2 million animal species and more than 0.5 million plants species have been identified and described.

As different there are so many species of living organisms on earth and they are known by different name in different geographical areas. Moreover the scientific community from the time of Aristotle always tried to develop a systemized method of classifying these species taking into account various parameters like, morphology, biochemical metabolic reactions and genetic evolution.

HISTORY AND TYPES OF CLASSIFICATION

1. **Artificial system of classification:** All taxonomists from Aristotle to Linnaeus, classified organisms on the basis of external observable (morphological) characters like floral structure (number of stamens), root modification, leaf venation, etc. In this system no weightage was given to natural and Phylogenetic relationship. Such system is based on one or a few superficial similarities. This is an arbitrary system of classification. Linnaeus also used such system of classification. This system may also be based upon habit and habitats of the organisms.

2. **Natural system classification:** It uses more number of characters and is based upon natural affinities using

homology and comparative study. Bentham-Hooker used this system of classification for angiosperms (seed producing plants).

3. **Numerical taxonomy (phenetics) or quantitative taxonomy:** This system uses numerical methods for evaluating the similarities and differences between the species. This uses maximum number of characters. This system uses computer analysis. This is known as **Adansonian system of classification** as it was first described by Adanson (1963).

4. **Phylogenetic classification (cladistics):** This system of classification is based upon evolutionary relationship and also uses morphological characters origin and evolution for classifying organisms. The family tree so found in this system is known as Cladogram. This classification was proposed by Hutchinson. A. Engler and K. Prantl published 'Phylogenetic system of classification' in plants.

5. **Karyotaxonomy:** This system of classification uses information like chromosome number, structure of chromosomes, size and shape of chromosomes and the behavior of chromosomes during meiosis.

6. **Chemotaxonomy:** This system is based on chemical products, particularly secondary metabolites.

7. **Experimental taxonomy:** In this classification relationship is determined by the genetics and breeding experiments.

8. **Biochemical taxonomy:** It is based on biochemistry of various chemicals like hormones and pheromones, etc.

9. **New systematics:** This covers systematic studies considering evolutionary relationship and other parameters like molecular biology, cytology, genetics, biochemistry, etc.

Scientific classification of plants is done by International Code of Botanical Nomenclature (ICBN) and for animals by International Code of Zoological Nomenclature (ICZN).

Basic Concepts of Taxonomic Hierarchy

There are seven basic categories of hierarchy:
1. Kingdom
2. Phylum (in animals)/division (in plants)
3. Class

4. Order
5. Family
6. Genus
7. Species

The term 'Taxon' is used to refer to any rank or level or category of the classification. Hence, the dogs, carnivora, mammals and animals are all taxa at different levels of hierarchy. The term 'taxon' for animals was given by Adolf Meyer (1926).

1. **Species:** It is the lowest category in basic taxonomic hierarchy and has the maximum common characteristics with other species under the same genus. In genus Panthera, there are several species.

2. **Genus:** The genus is an aggregate or a group of closely related species. The Taxon genus has more common characteristics with other genera than the higher ranks.

3. **Family:** It is the group of closely related genera, and has less common characteristics than species or genus rank.

4. **Order:** It is a higher taxon and is the assemblage of families having similar characteristics, however, the common characteristics will be fewer than at family or genus level. In mammals the common order is Primates.

5. **Class:** It is a group of related orders. The lizards, birds and cattle belong to class Reptilia.

6. **Phylum:** The classes with similar features are grouped into Phylum share very few common characteristics with other phyla. The common characteristics of phylum chordata are dorsal tubular nervous system. Notochord and the pharyngeal gill slits at some stage of life cycle. Other phyla are Annelida, Artropoda and Mollusca, etc.

7. **Kingdom:** The phyla are grouped into still broader categories called kingdom.

Thus in above taxonomic hierarchy as we move from lower to higher (species to kingdom) rank, the number of common characteristics go on decreasing. Lower the taxon more are the common characteristics and higher the taxon the fewer are the common features (Table 2.1).

Table 2.1 Example of taxonomy of humans

Common name	Biological name	Phylum	Class	Order	Family	Genus
Human	Homo sapiens	Chordate	Mamma-lia	Primates	Homi-nidae	Homo

BROAD CONCEPT OF CLASSIFICATION

There is a great diversity in structure, cellularity, habitat, mode of nutrition of different organisms in ecosystem. To understand these differences and similarities between different organisms, we can classify various animals and plants on the basis of the following parameters.

Cellularity

An organism can be unicellular or multicellular. The number of cells decides the structure, metabolic functions and other parameters of organisms. The characteristics of unicellular and multicellular are given in Table 2.2.

Table 2.2 Differences between unicellular and multicellular organisms

Characteristics	Unicellular organisms	Multicellular organisms
Cell number	Single cell	Large number of cells
Function	All functions are performed by single cell	Different cells perform different specific functions
Division of labor	Not performed	Cells specified to perform different functions
Reproduction	Involves the same single cell	Specialized cells, germ cells take part in reproduction
Life span	Short	Long

Ultra Structure: Prokaryotes or Eukaryotes

On the basis of internal structure of cell of an organism, cells can be divided into prokaryotes and eukaryotes. Characteristics of cell are given in Table 2.3 and Fig. 2.1.

Table 2.3   Differences between prokaryote and eukaryote

Prokaryotes	Eukaryotes
Circular DNA in cytosol	Linear DNA in nucleus
No organelles	Several membrane bound organelles
Nucleoid (not membrane bound)	Nucleus (membrane bound)
Single chromosome	Several chromosomes
Plasma membrane typically lack receptors	Plasma membrane with receptors
Chemically complex cell wall (may contain peptidoglycan)	Chemically simple cell walls
DNA transcription and mRNA translation occurs simultaneously	DNA transcription in nucleus and mRNA translation in cystol
Flagellum (if present) simple, built from two proteins	Flagellum (if present) complex, built from microtubules
May have pili and fimbriae	May have cilia
Haploid genome (only one copy of each gene)	Diploid genome (more than one copy of each gene)
May have plasmids (DNA outside chromosome)	Plasmid DNA not common
Compact genome (little repetitive DNA)	Usually large amounts of non-coding and repetitive DNA
May have a glycocalyx cover	Glycocalyx only if no cell wall
Small ribosomes	Large ribosomes in cystosol/nucleus small ribosomes in organelles
No histones in chromosomes	DNA 'wound' around histones
Lacks cytoskeleton	Cytoskeleton
Mycolaginous capsule	No mycolaginous capsule
Cell size range 0.5–100 mm	Cell size range 10–150 mm
Asexual reproduction	Sexual reproduction

Energy and Carbon Utilization

On the basis of energy and carbon utilization, the organism are divided into three types:

1. Autotrophs
2. Heterotrophs
3. Lithotropes

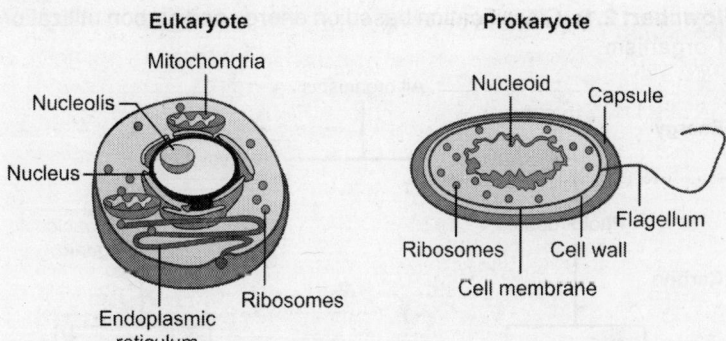

Fig. 2.1: Difference between prokaryote and eukaryote cells

Table 2.4 Classification based on energy and carbon utilization of organism

Microbial nutrition	
Carbon sources	
Autotrophs	CO_2 sole or principal biosynthetic carbon source
Heterotrophs	Reduced, performed, organic molecules from other organisms
Energy sources	
Phototrophs	Light
Chemotrophs	Oxidation of organic or inorganic compounds
Hydrogen and electron sources	
Lithotrophs	Reduced inorganic molecules
Organotrophs	Organic molecules

Phototrophs use light as an energy source, while chemotrophs use electron donors as a source of energy, whether from organic or inorganic sources; however, in the case of autotrophs, these electron donors come from inorganic chemical sources. Such chemotrophs are lithotrophs. An organism that eats other organism is called heterotrophy (Flowchart 2.1).

Roles and interactions of **Producers** (plants), **Consumers** (animals) and **Decomposers** (fungus, insects, etc). The **role** of a decomposer is to decompose or break down dead matter in the environment. Plants make their own food by the process of photosynthesis and also produce food for other **consumers**. Without **producers** an **ecosystem** could not sustain itself.

Flowchart 2.1: Classification based on energy and carbon utilization of organism

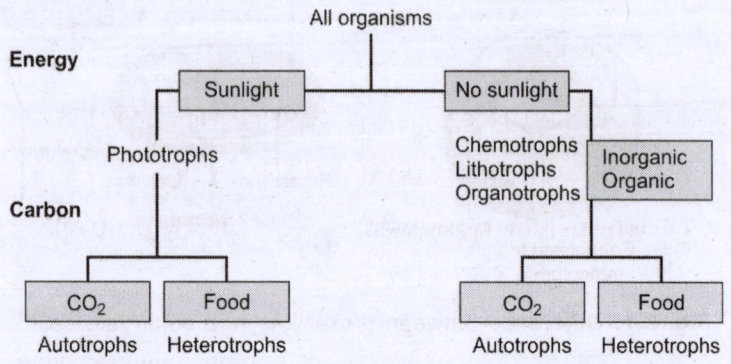

1. Herbivores—eat only producers
2. Carnivores—eat only other consumers
3. Omnivores—eat both producers and consumers

Ammonia Excretion

1. Animals can also be divided on the basis of their excretory material which is related to their habitat and body metabolism. There is no general pathway for nitrogen excretion in plants. The major excretory material in animal is nitrogen. In animals it is not directly excreted but through formation of various compounds. On the basis of excretion animals can be divided into 3 types (Table 2.5).

2. Ammonotelic animals excrete amino nitrogen as ammonia (most aquatic species, such as the bony fishes).

3. Ureotelic animals excrete amino nitrogen in the form of urea (most terrestrial animals).

4. Uricotelic animals excrete amino nitrogen as uric acid (birds and reptiles).

Habitat: Aquatic or Terrestrial

On the basis of habitat which means the ideal place of growth and expansion of animals and plants in an ecosystem. The animals and plants can be classified into aquatic and terrestrial forms (Table 2.6).

Table 2.5 Classification based on ammonia excretion

Waste	Advantages	Disadvantages	Habitat	Excreted by
Ammonia	Produced with little energy	Toxic in conc. solution. Requires a lot of water for excretion.	Water	Marine and fresh water invertebrates, bony fish, amphibian
Urea	Less toxic than ammonia, requires less water for excretion	Requires little more energy to produce it	Land, sea	Adult amphibians, turtles, mammals
Uric acid	Very little water is required for excretion	Requires considerable energy to produce it	Land	Reptiles, birds, insects, land gastro pods

Characteristics of aquatic and terrestrial animals

Table 2.6 Differences between aquatic and terrestrial animals

Aquatic animals	Terrestrial animals
An aquatic is an animal who lives in water	A terrestrial animal is an animal who lives exclusively in the land
Respire through gills and their skin	Respire through lungs or trachea
Show adaptations such as streamline bodies, fins, webbed feet and air bladder	Show adaptations such as legs, waterproof skin, feathers, covered eggs and kidneys
Skin is slimy, slippery and soft	Skin is leathery, hard and spiny

Characteristics of Aquatic and Terrestrial Plants

1. **Terrestrial plants:** The plants that grow on the land are called terrestrial trees. Examples are rubber tree and teak tree. Smaller plants like sugarcane, rice, cotton, pepper also grow here.
2. **Aquatic plants:** Underwater plants. These have narrow leaves without any stomata. They breathe through water and clean it. Examples are tape grass, pond weed, etc.

MOLECULAR BASIS OF CLASSIFICATION OF ORGANISMS

Carl Woese et al. classified organisms into three domain classification based on sequence of ribosomal RNA genes and formed the molecular basis of dividing all organisms into six kingdoms.

3 Domains and 6 Kingdoms Classification

I Domain Bacteria

1. **Kingdom Eubacteria:** Unicellular and prokaryotic with peptidoglycan

II Domain Archaea

2. **Kingdom Archaea:** Unicellular and prokaryotic without peptidoglycan

III Domain Eukarya

3. **Kingdom Protista:** Unicellular/multicellular and eukaryotic
4. **Kingdom Fungi:** Unicellular/multicellular, eukaryotic and decomposers
5. **Kingdom Plantae:** Multicellular, eukaryotic and autotrophic
6. **Kingdom Animalia:** Multicellular, eukaryotic and hetero-trophic

Model Organisms

A model organism is a species that has been widely studied, usually because it is easy to maintain and breed in a laboratory setting and has particular experimental advantages. Organisms that have been widely used for research so that a great deal is known about their biology. These organisms have properties that made them excellent research subjects (Table 2.7).

The characteristics of model organisms are:

1. Relatively easy to grow and maintain in a restricted space
2. Relatively short generation time (birth → reproduction → birth)
3. Relatively well understood growth and development

4. Relatively easy to provide necessary nutrients for growth

5. Closely resemble other organisms or systems

Table 2.7 Different types of model organism

Genetic model organisms	Experimental model organisms	Genomic model organisms
Good candidates for genetic analysis	Good candidates for research in developmental biology	Good candidate for genome research
Breed in large numbers. Have short generation time, hence large scale crosses can be followed over several generations. Example: Drosophila	Produce robust embryos that can be easily manipulated and studied. Example: Frog	Easy to manage genomes, e.g. small genomes size or limited number of repeats. Genome is similar to a human Example: Rat

1. **Mammalian models:**
   - Mouse (*Mus musculus)*
   - Rat (*Rattus norvegicus*)

2. **Non-mammalian models**
   - Bacterium (*Escherichia coli*)
   - Baker's or brewer's yeast (*Saccharomyces cerevisiae*)
   - *Nematode* (*Caenorhabditis elegans*)
   - Fruit fly (*Drosophila melanogaster*)
   - Zebra fish (*Danio rerio*)

3. **Plant model**
   - *Arabidopsis thaliana*

E. coli

It is a natural mammalian gut bacteria used as model organism because of its simplicity it has been the favoured organism for studying fundamental aspects of biochemistry and molecular biology. Most of our present concepts of molecular biology—DNA replication, genetic code, gene expression and protein synthesis come from the study of *E. coli*. Some reasons to make *E. coli* model organism are:

1. *E. coli* is a single-celled organism so it is simple to study.

2. Its life cycle is short.

3. It can easily grow on nutrient medium.

4. It can be easily genetically manipulated.

Mouse (Mus Musculus)

The mouse has developed into the premier mammalian model system for genetic research. Scientists from a wide range of biomedical fields have gravitated to the mouse because of its close genetic and physiological similarities to humans, as well as the ease with which its genome can be manipulated and analyzed. Some of the reasons to make mouse as the model organism are:

1. These are small, maintained easily and have a short life span.

2. All new drugs, treatments are tried on mice.

3. Their genetics, biological characters resemble humans.

Fruit Fly (Drosophila melanogaster)

The fruit fly *Drosophila melanogaster* is a versatile model organism that has been used in biomedical research for over a century to study a broad range of phenomena. There are many technical advantages of using *Drosophila* over vertebrate:

1. Relationship between humans genes and fruit fly genes is close.

2. Seventy-five percent of genes that cause human diseases are found in fruit fly.

3. They have a short life span—(8–14) days.

4. These are inexpensive to maintain.

5. These have a simple diet needing some carbohydrates and some proteins.

6. It is easy to manipulate genes in fruit fly.

Yeast (Saccharomyces cerevisiae)

Yeast is one of the simplest eukaryotic organisms but many essential cellular processes are the same in yeast and humans. It is therefore an important organism to study to understand the basic molecular processes in humans.

Baker's or budding yeast has long been a popular model organism for basic biological research because of the following reasons:

1. It is easy to manipulate in the lab.
2. Yeast can cope with a variety of environmental conditions.
3. Yeast shows cell division in a similar way to our cells. In 1996, it was the first eukaryotic organism to have its genome sequenced.
4. Twenty percent of genes causing diseases are found in yeast.
5. Many drugs are tested on yeast which have functional equivalent of mutated human genes to reverse the disease.

Nematode (Caenorhabditis Elegans)

At approximately 1 mm in length and transparent, the nematode worm might seem an unusual choice of animal to study in such detail. But this peculiar soil-dwelling roundworm has proved itself to be a vital research tool. In fact, it is arguably the single most described animal in scientific literature because of the following reasons:

1. It can easily grow in labs on nutrient medium.
2. It produces over thousand eggs each day.
3. Worm is transparent so its cells can be easily studied.
4. Its development (molecular signals) is found in complex organisms like humans, so it is easy to study nervous system of higher organisms.
5. Its genes can be easily mutated.
6. Many genes have functional counterparts in humans so diseases can be easily studied.

A. thaliana (Arabidopsis thaliana)

A. thaliana is a small flowering plant that is widely used as a model organism in plant biology. Arabidopsis is a member of the mustard (Brassicaceae) family, which includes cultivated species such as cabbage and radish. Arabidopsis is not of major agronomic significance, but it offers important advantages for basic research in genetics and molecular biology. It is used as a model organism because of the following reasons:

1. It has a small genome (114.5 Mb/125 Mb total) has been sequenced in the year 2000.
2. It has a short life span of about six weeks.
3. It can be easily cultivated.
4. Mutations can be easily produced in this plant.

KEY POINTS

- Nomenclature: It is the process of giving scientific names (not vernacular or local names) to the organisms.
- Classification: It is the process of grouping animals and plants into convenient categories on the basis of certain observable traits.
- Identification: It is determination of correct position of an organism in the classification.
- Taxonomy: It is the study of the process of classification.
- Systematic: This includes the identification, nomenclature and classification of organisms based on various parameters.
- Hippocrates: He classified animals into various groups like insects, fishes and birds, etc.
- Aristotle: Known as father of zoology/biology. He had written Historia animalium.
- Theophrastus: Known as father of botany
- John Ray—(1686): A British botanist.
- Carrolus Linnaeus: A Swedish naturalist—father of taxonomy. He coined the terms 'class' and 'systematics'.
- The basic unit of biological classification is known as species which is defined as group of natural population of animals and plants, whose members can interbreed among themselves.
- The seven basic categories of taxonomic hierarchy are:
  1. Kingdom
  2. Phylum (in animals)/division (in plants)

3. Class
4. Order
5. Family
6. Genus
7. Species

- The term 'Taxon' is used to refer to any rank or level or category of the classification. Hence, the dogs, carnivora, mammals and animals are all taxa at different levels of hierarchy.
- Genus: The genus is an aggregate or a group of closely related species.
- Family: It is the group of closely related genera
- Order: It is a higher taxon and is the assemblage of families having similar characteristics.
- Class: It is a group of related orders. Examples are lizards, birds and cattle belong to class Reptilia.
- Phylum: The classes with similar features are grouped into Phylum
- Kingdom: The phyla are grouped into still broader categories called kingdom.
- Cellularity: An organism can be unicellular or multi-cellular.
- On the basis of energy and carbon utilization the organisms are divided into three types:
  1. Autotrophs
  2. Heterotrophs
  3. Lithotrophs
- Phototrophs use light as an energy source, while chemo-trophs use electron donors as a source of energy.
- Heterotrophs: An organism that eats other organism.
- Herbivores: Eat only producers.
- Carnivores: Eat only other consumers.
- Omnivores: Eat both producers and consumers.
- Ammonotelic animals excrete amino nitrogen as ammonia (most aquatic species, such as the bony fishes).

- Ureotelic animals excrete amino nitrogen in the form of urea (most terrestrial animals).
- Uricotelic animals excrete amino nitrogen as uric acid (birds and reptiles).
- Terrestrial plants: The plants that grow on the land are called terrestrial trees. Example is rubber tree.
- Aquatic plants: Underwater plants. They breathe through water and clean it. Example is pond weed.
- Carl Woese et al. classified organisms into 3 domain classification based on sequence of ribosomal RNA genes.
- *E. coli*: It is a natural mammalian gut bacteria
- The fruit fly *Drosophila melanogaster* is a versatile model organism—used in biomedical research—have many technical advantages
- Yeast (*Saccharomyces cerevisiae*) *Yeast is one of the simplest eukaryotic organisms—important organism to study to understand basic molecular processes in humans.*
- *A. thaliana* is a small flowering plant that is widely used as a model organism in plant biology.

PRACTICE QUESTIONS

Very Short Answer Type Questions

1. Who is the father of zoology?
2. Who is the father of botany?
3. What is a model organism?
4. Who introduced 5 kingdoms classification?
5. What are prokaryotes?
6. What are eukaryotes?
7. What are autotrophs?
8. Who is the father of taxonomy?
9. What is the scientific name of fruit fly?
10. Give one example of simplest eukaryotic organism.

Short Answer Type Questions

1. What is taxonomy?
2. What is classification?
3. What is nomenclature?
4. What is dominance?
5. Explain the term: (a) Species, (b) genus, (c) family, (d) order, (e) class, (f) phylum, (g) kingdom.
6. Give any two differences between (a) prokaryotes and eukaryotes, (b) autotrophs and heterotrophs, (c) ureotelic and uricotelic.

Long Answer Type Questions

1. What is the role of nomenclature in taxonomy?
2. Explain the concept of taxonomic hierarchy.
3. Explain the classification of organisms based on carbon utilization of organism.
4. Explain how did Carl Woese classified organisms.
5. What are the characteristics of model organisms?
6. Explain the use of mouse, *E. coli*, yeast fruit fly as model organisms.

Genetics

COMMON TERMS USED IN GENETICS

1. Genetics is the study of inheritance and variation.
2. Term genetics was first used by W. Bateson 1905.
3. Gregor Johann Mendel is called father of genetics
4. Heredity or inheritance is the process by which character are passed on from parent to progeny.
5. Variation is the characteristics difference by which progeny differs from their parents.
6. Cause of variation is sexual reproduction.
7. *Phenotype:* External appearance or trait of an individual
8. *Genotype:* Genetic constitution of an organism
9. *Genes or mendelian factor:* Units of inheritance. They contain information required to express a particular trait

10. *Alleles or allelmorphs:* The two Mendelian factors or gene which occur on the same locus in two homologous chromosomes of an individual and control the expression of a character called allels or allelomorphs or alternative form of same gene, e.g. T and t, Y and y, R and r are pair alleles.

11. *Dominant factor of allele:* It is one allele of the allele pair which can express itself whether present in homozygous or heterozygous state is called dominant allele, e.g. the factor for tallness in hybrid and homogenous states Tt and TT can express itself.

12. *Recessive factor or allele:* The factor of an allelic or allelomorphic pair which is unable to express its effect in the presence of its contrasting factor in heterozygous state is called recessive factor of allele. A recessive allele is represented by small letter, e.g. in Tt. The effect of recessive factor becomes known only when it is present in the pure or homozygous state, e.g. tt in dwarf pea plant

13. *Hybrid:* The heterozygous organism produced after crossing of genetically different individuals is called hybrid.

14. *Homozygous:* Both alleles are same/similar for a character e.g. TT = tall, tt = dwarf.

15. *Genome:* It is a complete set of chromosomes where every gene and chromosome is represented singly as in a gamete.

16. *Gene pool:* The aggregate of all the genes and their alleles presents in an interbreeding population is known as a gamete.

17. *Punnett square:* It is a graphical representation to calculate the probability of all genotypes of offsprings in a genetic cross. RC Punnett introduced Punnett square (in 1972) to figure out the probable result of genetic cross. The following points must be kept in mind when constructing the Punnett square:

   a. A letter represents a character, e.g. T and t represent character of plant height.

   b. A capital letter, e.g. T represents a dominant character or allele.

   c. A small or lower case letter, e.g. t represents the recessive character or trait.

   d. Paired letter represents the genotype.

INTRODUCTION TO GENETICS

Genetics is a branch of biology concerned with the study of genes, genetic variation, and heredity in living organisms.

Or

Genetics is the study of heredity and how qualities and characteristics are passed on from one generation to another by means of genes.

Gregor Johann Mendel conducted hybridisation experiments on garden pea (*Pisum sativum*) for seven years (1856–1863) and proposed the laws of inheritance in living organisms. He is also known as Father of Genetics.

Mendel experimental material: He selected garden pea plant as a sample for the following reasons:

1. Pea is available in many varieties on a large scale to observe alternate traits.
2. Peas are self-pollinated and can be cross-pollinated also to prevent self-pollination.
3. These are annual plants with a short life cycle. So, several generations can be studied within a short period.
4. Pea plants could easily be raised, maintained and handled.
5. Many varieties are available with distinct characteristics. Which plants provide many easily detectable contrasting characters.

Mendel conducted artificial pollination/cross-pollination experiments using several true-breeding pea lines. A true-breeding line refers to one that have undergone continuous self-pollination and showed stable trait inheritance and expression for several generations. Mendel selected 14 true-breeding pea plant varieties, as pair, which were similar except for one character with contrasting traits.

Mendel's Law

Mendel's laws of inheritance are based on his observations on monohybrid crosses.

He proposed the following laws of inheritance:

Principle of Dominance

The principle of dominance states that when two alternative forms of a trait or character (genes) are present in an organism, only one factor expresses itself in F1-progeny and is called dominant, while the other that remains masked is called recessive.

This law is used to explain the expression of only one of the parental characters in a monohybrid cross in the F1-generation and the expression of both in the F2-generation. It also explains the proportion of 3:1 obtained in the F2-generation (Fig. 3.1).

Law of Segregation (First Law)

This law states that the alleles do not show any blending and both the characters are recovered as such in the F2-generation, though one of these is not seen in the F1-generation.

Due to this, the gametes are pure for a character. The parents contain two alleles during gamete formation.

The factors or alleles of a pair segregate from each other such that a gamete receives only one of the two factors (Fig. 3.1).

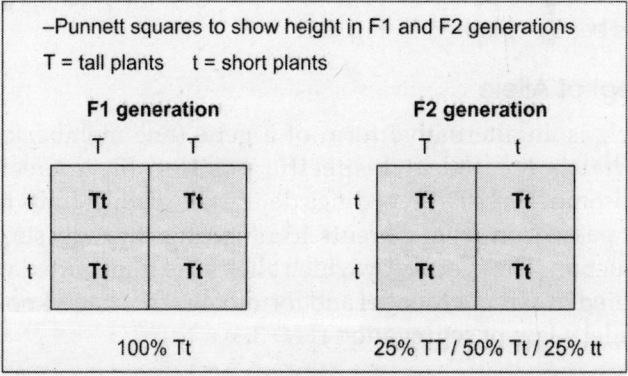

Fig. 3.1: Punnett square showing law of segregation

Mendel discovered that, when he crossed tall pea plant with dwarf pea plant the result was in the F1 generation (offspring) all tall pea plants were produced. When Mendel self-fertilized the F1 generation pea plants, he obtained tall pea plants to dwarf pea plants ratio in the F2 generation of 3:1.

Law of Independent Assortment *(Second Law)*

This law states that when two pairs of traits are combined in a hybrid, segregation of one pair of character is independent of the other pair of characters at the time of gamete formation.

It also gets randomly rearranged in the offsprings producing both parental and new combinations of characters. The law was proposed by Mendel, based on the results of dihybrid crosses, where inheritance of two traits were considered simultaneously.

Mendel performed di-hybrid cross in pea plants that were true breeding for two traits, for example, a plant that had round seeds and yellow seed color was cross pollinated with a plant that had wrinkled seed and green seed color.

In this cross, the traits for round seed (RR) and yellow seed color (YY) are dominant. Wrinkled seed (rr) and green seed color (yy) are recessive. The resulting offspring F1 generation were all heterozygous for round seed and yellow color (RrYy). This means the dominant traits of round seed shaped and yellow color completely masked the recessive traits in F1 generation.

Mendel allowed the F1 plants to self pollinate, thus in F2 generation he noticed a ratio of (9:3: 3:1) in the phenotypes, this has been explained in Fig. 3.2.

Concept of Allele

An allele is an alternative form of a gene (one member of a pair) that is located at a specific position on a specific chromosome. These DNA codings determine distinct traits that can be passed on from parents to offspring through sexual reproduction. The process by which alleles are transmitted was discovered by Gregor Mendel and formulated in what is known as Mendel's law of segregation (Fig. 3.3).

Examples of Dominant and Recessive Alleles

Diploid organisms typically have two alleles for a trait.

When allele pairs are the same, they are homozygous. When the alleles of a pair are heterozygous, the phenotype of one trait may be dominant and the other recessive. The dominant allele is expressed and the recessive allele is masked. This is

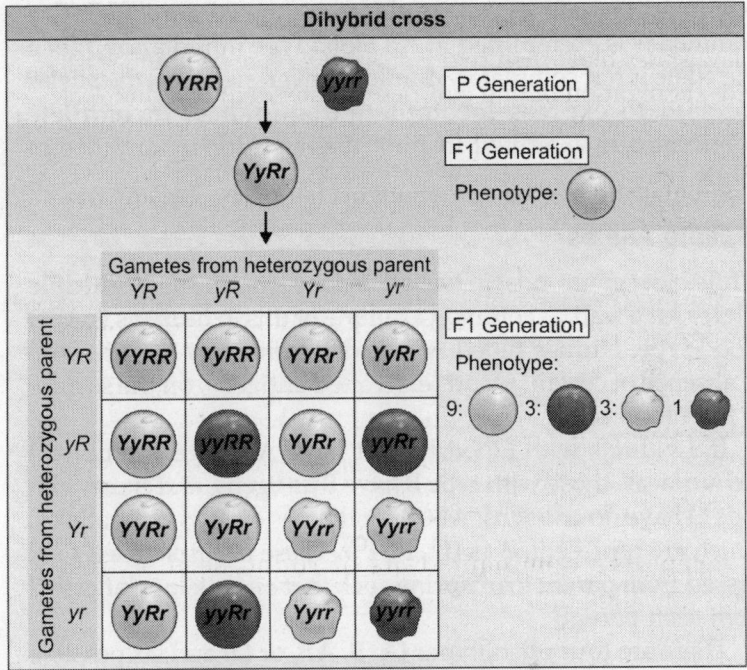

Fig. 3.2: Law of independent assortment

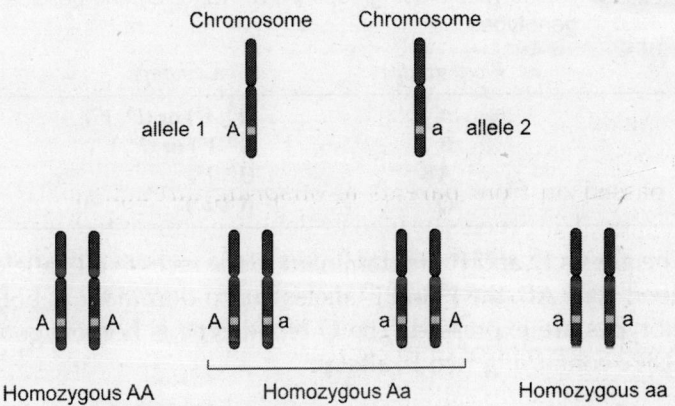

Fig. 3.3: Chromosomes and alleles

known as complete dominance. In heterozygous relationships where neither allele is dominant but both are completely expressed, the alleles are considered to be co-dominant. Co-dominance is exemplified in AB blood type inheritance. When one allele is not completely dominant over the other, the alleles are said to express incomplete dominance. Incomplete dominance is exhibited in pink flower color inheritance in tulips.

Multiple Alleles

While most genes exist in two allele forms, some have **multiple alleles** for a trait. A common example of this in humans is ABO blood type. Human blood type is determined by the presence or absence of certain identifiers, called antigens, on the surface of red blood cells.

Individuals with blood type A have A antigens on blood cell surfaces, those with type B have B antigens, and those with type O have no antigens. ABO blood types exist as three alleles, which are represented as (I^A, I^B, I^O). These multiple alleles are passed from parent to offspring such that one allele is inherited from each parent.

There are four phenotypes **(A, B, AB, or O)** and six possible genotypes for human ABO blood groups (Table 3.1).

Table 3.1 Phenotypes blood groups (A, B, AB, or O) and possible genotypes

S.No	Blood groups	Genotype
1	A	(I^A, I^A) or (I^A, I^O)
2	B	(I^B, I^B) or (I^B, I^O)
3	AB	(I^A, I^B)
4	O	(I^O, I^O)

The alleles I^A and I^B are dominant to the recessive I^O allele. In blood type AB, the I^A and I^B alleles are co-dominant as both phenotypes are expressed. The O blood type is homozygous recessive containing two I^O alleles.

Gene Mapping

Also called linkage mapping—can offer firm evidence that a disease transmitted from parent to child is linked to one or more genes. Mapping also provides clues about which chromosome contains the gene and precisely where the gene lies on that chromosome.

A map of where the genes are in relationship to each other on the chromosomes can then be drawn. This is called a linkage map. Genes that are on the same chromosome are said to be 'linked' and the distance between these genes is called a 'linkage distance'.

To produce a genetic map, researchers collect blood or tissue samples from members of families in which a certain disease or trait is prevalent, DNA markers don't, by themselves, identify the gene responsible for the disease or trait; but they can tell researchers roughly where the gene is on the chromosome. Gene mapping is divided into two forms, i.e. chromosome mapping and DNA mapping.

DNA mapping is done by determining a DNA sequence to a specific chromosome. It can be done by various techniques like,

1. Chromosome jumping
2. Pulsed feel gel electrophoresis
3. Gene cloning

Genetic Mapping

Genetic mapping—also called linkage mapping—can offer firm evidence that a disease transmitted from parent to child is linked to one or more genes. Mapping also provides clues about which chromosome contains the gene and precisely where the gene lies on that chromosome.

Genetic maps have been used successfully to find the gene responsible for relatively rare, single gene inherited disorders such as cystic fibrosis and Duchenne muscular dystrophy. Genetic maps are also useful in guiding scientists to the many genes that are believed to play a role in the development of more common disorders such as asthma, heart disease, diabetes, cancer, and psychiatric conditions.

Procedure of Producing Genetic Map

To produce a genetic map, researchers collect blood or tissue samples from members of families in which a certain disease or trait is prevalent. Using various laboratory techniques, the scientists isolate DNA from these samples and examine it for unique patterns that are seen only in family members who have the disease or trait. These characteristic patterns in the chemical bases that make up DNA are referred to as DNA markers.

Genetic Markers

Markers themselves usually consist of DNA that does not contain a gene. But because markers can help a researcher locate a disease-causing gene, they are extremely valuable for tracking inheritance of traits through generations of a family.

Genome Mapping

Genetic mapping is based on the use of genetic techniques to construct maps showing the positions of genes and other sequence features on a genome. Genetic techniques include cross breeding experiments and in case of humans, the examination of family histories (pedigrees).

Physical mapping uses molecular biology techniques to examine DNA molecules directly in order to construct maps showing the positions of sequence features, including genes.

Physical Mapping

Restriction mapping, which locates the relative positions on a DNA molecule of the recognition sequences for restriction endonucleases. Fluorescent *in situ* hybridization (FISH), in which marker locations are mapped by hybridizing a probe containing the marker to intact chromosomes

Sequence tagged site (STS) mapping, in which the positions of short sequences are mapped by PCR and/or hybridization analysis of genome fragments. Example explaining the genetic map (Fig. 3.4). Genes are shown in relative orders and distance from each other based on pedigree studies

The chance of the chromosome breaking between A and C is higher than the chance of the chromosome breaking between A and B during meiosis. Similarly, the chance of the chromosome breaking between E and F is higher than the chance of

Genetic maps

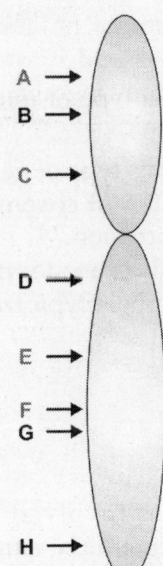

A →
B →

C →

D →

E →

F →
G →

H →

• Genes are shown in relative order and distance from each other based on pedigree studies.

• The chance of the chromosome breaking between A and C is higher than the chance of the chromosome breaking between A and B during meiosis.

• Similarly, the chance of the chromosome breaking between C and F is higher than the chance of the chromosome breaking F and G.

• The closer two genes are, the more likely they are to be inherited together (co-occurrence)

• If pedigree studies show a high incidence of co-occurrence, those genes will be located close together on a genetic map.

Fig. 3.4: Explanation of genetic mapping

the chromosome breaking between F and G. The closer two genes are, the more likely they are to be inherited together (co-occurrence). If pedigree studies show a high incidence of co-occurrence, those genes will be located close together on a genetic map.

GENE INTERACTION

Definition

The phenomenon of two or more genes affecting the expression of each other in various ways in the development of a single character of an organism is known as gene interaction.

Most of the characters of living organisms are controlled/influenced/governed by a collaboration of several different genes. Mendel and other workers assumed that characters are governed by single genes but later it was discovered that many characters are governed by two or more genes.

Types of Gene Interactions

Gene interaction can be classified as:

1. **Allelic/non-epistatic gene interaction:** This type of interaction gives the classical ratio of 3:1 or 9:3:3:1.

2. **Non-allelic/epistatic gene interaction:** In this type of gene interaction genes located on same or different chromosomes interact with each other for their expression.

   Discovery of non-allelic gene interaction has been made after Mendel and can be understood by studying phenotypic trait of gene.

   Gene interaction can be of the following types:

Complementary Gene Interaction

1. Involves two pairs of non-allelic genes

2. When dominant forms of both the genes involved in complementary gene interaction are alone have same phenotypic expression.

3. But, if they are present in combination, yield different phenotypic effect.

4. Flower color in garden pea follows this type of gene interaction.

We have considered garden pea for the explanation of this type of gene interaction, in which it was noted for the first time. Two different varieties of garden pea produce same color flowers—white. But on crossing they yield purple color flowers. Again in F2, 9 purple : 7 white segregation was observed.

Supplementary Gene Interaction

1. Involves two pairs of non-allelic genes

2. Affect the same character

3. One of the dominant genes has visible effect itself.

4. Second dominant gene expresses itself when supplemented by the other dominant gene of a pair.

5. Coat color (black, albino and agouti) of mice follows supplementary gene interaction.

In mice, black coat color is monogenetically dominant over albino and agouti. The offspring resulting from the cross between black and albino has agouti coat color.

F2 generation shows segregation in the ratio 9 agouti: 3 black: 4 albino. This behavior is based on ratio of dihybrid cross, so the trait must be governed by two pairs of genes.

Suppose, gene C is essential for the development of black coat color, so present in black mice and absent in albino mice. Albino mice contains only gene A, so produces albino phenotype.

But, when gene A is present along with gene C, produces agouti phenotype. Both the genes in recessive form produce albino phenotype.

So the cross will be as follows:

Cross between	F1	F2
CCaa X ccAAblack X albino	CcAa agouti	9 agouti: 3 black: 4 albino

Incomplete Dominance

Incomplete dominance is a form of intermediate inheritance in which one allele for a specific trait is not completely expressed over its paired allele. This results in a third phenotype in which the expressed physical trait is a combination of the phenotypes of both alleles. Unlike complete dominance inheritance, one allele does not dominate or mask the other.

Incomplete dominance occurs in the polygenic inheritance of traits such as eye color and skin color.

Discovery of no allelic gene interaction has been made after Mendel and can be understood by studying phenotypic trait of gene.

EPISTASIS

Definition

Suppression of the effect of a gene by another gene. One gene completely masks another gene. For example, coat color in mice

= 2 separate genes, C, c – pigment (C) or no pigment (c) and B, b – more pigment (black = B) or less (brown= b), cc = albino, no matter B allele (Fig. 3.5).

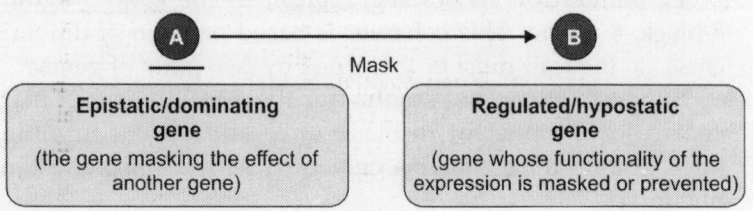

Fig. 3.5: Gene interaction

Mitosis and Meiosis

Cells divide and reproduce in two ways—mitosis and meiosis.

Mitosis is a process of cell division that results in two genetically identical daughter cells developing from a single parent cell.

Meiosis, on the other hand, is the division of a germ cell involving two fissions of the nucleus and giving rise to four gametes, or sex cells, each possessing half the number of chromosomes of the original cell (Table 3.2).

How Genetic Material Passes from Parents to Offspring

The genetic information passed from parent to offspring is contained in genes carried by chromosomes in the nucleus. Sexual reproduction produces offspring that resemble their parents, but are not identical to them.

Genetic Information

Offspring resemble their parents because they contain genetic information passed on to them by their parents.

Chromosomes and Genes

Chromosomes, found in the *cell nucleus*, contain many genes. A gene is a section of *DNA*, which carries coding for a particular *protein*. Different genes control the development of different characteristics of an organism. Many genes are needed to carry all the genetic information for a whole organism (Fig. 3.6).

Table 3.2 Comparison chart meiosis versus mitosis

	Meiosis	*Mitosis*
Definition	Type of cellular reproduction in which the number of chromosomes are reduced by half through the separation of homologous chromosomes, producing two haploid cells.	Process of asexual reproduction in which the cell divides in two producing a replica, with an equal number of chromosomes in each resulting diploid cell.
Type of reproduction	Sexual	Asexual
Occurs in	Humans, animals, plants.	All organisms.
Crossing over	Yes, mixing of chromosomes can occur.	No, crossing over cannot occur.
Chromosome number	Reduced by half.	Remains the same.
Steps	(Meiosis 1) Prophase I, Metaphase I, Anaphase I, Telophase I; (Meiosis 2) Prophase II, Metaphase II, Anaphase II and Telophase II.	Prophase, Metaphase, Anaphase, Telophase.
Creates	Sex cells only: female egg cells or male sperm cells.	Makes everything other than sex cells.
Function	Genetic diversity through sexual reproduction.	Cellular reproduction and general growth and repair of the body.

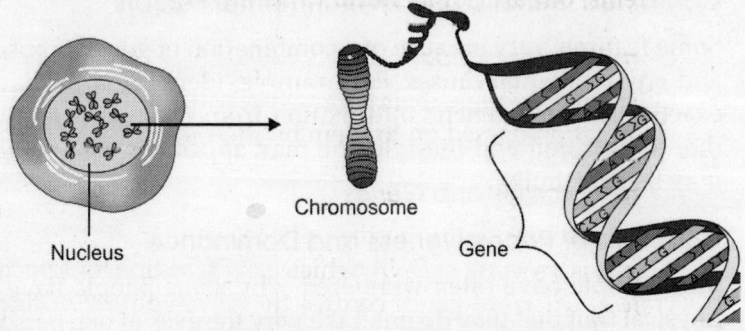

Nucleus

Chromosome

Gene

Fig. 3.6: Nucleus, chromosome and gene

Genetic Factors

The individuals of a species may look similar but they are not usually identical, these differences are called **variation**.

Inherited Variation

Variation due to **genetic causes** is inherited variation. For example, children usually look a little like their father, and a little like their mother, but they will not be identical to either of their parents. This is because they get half of their inherited features from each parent. Here are some examples of inherited variation

1. Eye color
2. Hair color
3. Skin color.

Environmental Variation

Some variation within a species is inherited, and some variation is due to the environment; some variation is due to a **combination** of both. Characteristics of animal and plant species can be affected by environmental factors like

1. Climate
2. Diet
3. Culture
4. Lifestyle, for example, one who eats too much will become heavier.

Combined Genetic and Environmental Factors

Some features vary because of a combination of genetic causes and environmental causes. For example, identical twins have exactly the same genetic information from their parents. But due to nutrition and lifestyle one may appear fit while other may become bulky.

Concepts of Recessiveness and Dominance

Most people have often wondered why some people have a physical trait that they do not. Like why the eyes of one person is blue and other are deep brown. These differences are caused by genes, which all contain specific information. Everyone inherits two copies of each gene from their parents, and the copies can either be different or the same. If the copies are different, then one is going to mask the effects of the other. The gene that trumps over the other is usually known as the **dominant gene**, and the weaker gene is known as **recessive**. In the presence of a dominant gene, a recessive gene will not show its traits. When two recessive genes are paired their traits will be visible. Dominant genes are also the ones whose traits are visible in the offspring. For recessive traits to be visible, both parents have to carry that recessive gene singly or in a pair.

Genes are usually termed dominant or recessive for a number of reasons. It is first important to note that genes are simply an instruction manual that is used to make certain protein. The protein made is what is actually responsible for the traits that are presented physically, like red hair or blue eyes. Since there are two copies of each gene (courtesy of both the parents), the 'instruction manual' in the mother's genes may be slightly different from the one in the father. The combination of these two sets of instructions will cause the formation of a slightly different protein. The reason why some genes are dominant and other recessive all lies in the making of the proteins. When a gene makes a protein that is functional, then that gene is dominant. If the protein formed is broken, then the gene that has formed is recessive.

A good example of this is the occurrence of red hair, which happens when a crucial protein in hair pigmentation fails to convert the red pigment to black, thus causing a build up of the former. If this protein is even slightly functional, then the person will not have red hair. This is where the concept of dominant and recessive genes is derived.

Pedigree characteristics of autosomal recessive, autosomal dominant, X-linked recessive, X-linked dominant and Y-linked traits.

Autosomal Recessive Traits

1. Appears in both sexes with equal frequency
2. Trait tends to skip generations

3. Affected offspring are usually born unaffected parents.

4. When both parents are heterozygous, approximately ¼ of the offspring will be affected.

5. Appears more frequently among the children of consanguine marriages.

Autosomal Dominant Trait

1. Appears in both sexes with equal frequency

2. Both sexes transmit the trait to their offspring

3. Does not skip generations

4. Affected offspring must have an affected parent, unless they possess a new mutations

5. When one parent is affected (heterozygous) and the other parent is unaffected, approximately ½ of the offspring will be affected

6. Unaffected parents do not transmit the trait.

X-linked Recessive Trait

1. More males than females are affected

2. Affected sons are usually born to unaffected mothers; thus, the trait skips generations.

3. A carrier (heterozygous) mother produces approximately ½ affected sons.

4. Is never passed from father to son.

5. All daughters of affected fathers are carriers.

X-linked Dominant Trait

1. Both males and females are affected; often more females than males are affected.

2. Does not skip generations. Affected sons must have an affected mother; affected daughters must have either an affected mother or an affected father.

3. Affected fathers will pass the trait on to all their daughters.

4. Affected mothers (if heterozygous) will pass the trait on to ½ of their sons and ½ of their daughters.

Y-linked Trait

1. Only males are affected
2. Is passed to all sons from father
3. Does not skip generations.

CONCEPT OF MAPPING OF PHENOTYPE TO GENES

Genotype vs. Phenotype

Genotype

The genetic makeup of an organism; the gene (or allele) combination an organism has. Example: Tt, ss GG, Ww.

Phenotype

The physical characteristics of an organism. The way an organism looks. For example: Curly hair, straight hair, blue eyes, tall.

Single Gene Disorders in Humans

Single gene disorders are caused by DNA changes in one particular gene, and often have predictable inheritance patterns. Over 10,000 human disorders are caused by a change, known as a mutation in a single gene. These are known as single gene disorders. The mutated version of the gene responsible for the disorder is known as a mutant, or disease, allele. Single gene disorders can be divided into different categories like dominant, recessive and X-linked (Table 3.3).

Single Gene Disorder

Gene mutation in autosomes:

1. **Recessively inherited trails:** These are caused by recessive genes in homozygous conditions. Some examples are:
   i. *Alkaptonuria:* It is caused by disorder in single gene. The symptom may include blackening of urine on exposure to O_2 and darkening of cartilages.
   ii. *Albinism:* It is caused by lack of pigment melanin in skin, hair and iris of eye. It is caused by absence of enzyme tyrosinase which produces melanin. It is seen when both the alleles of gene are recessive.

Table 3.3 Types of inheritance with characteristics and examples

Type of inheritance	Characteristics	Examples
Autosomal dominant	Both sexes equally affected: Vertical transmission	Huntington disease Achondroplasia NF
	Father to son transmission	Marfan syndrome
	Affected individuals transmit trait to ~ 50% offspring	
Autosomal recessive	Both sexes equally affected. Usually no prior family history	Hurler syndrome Cystic fibrosis Sickle cell anemia
	Consanguinity	Phenylketonuria (PKU)
	Mating between two carriers transmits trait to ~ 25% offspring	β-thalassemia

iii. *Sickle cell anemia:* It is autosomal recessive disease so it is transmitted from parents to offspring when both parents are carrier (heterozygote) for the gene. The disease is controlled by single pair of allels Hb^A and Hb^S. Three gene types are possible.

 a. $Hb^A Hb^A$ (Normal)

 b. $Hb^A Hb^S$ (Carrier)

 c. $Hb^S Hb^S$ (Disease)

This disease is caused when glutamic acid is replaced by valine.

Thalassemia: It is autosomal recessive disease. It is caused by defect in synthesis of globin polypeptide in RBC resulting in severe anemia.

X-linked Inheritance

X-linked inheritance means that the gene causing the trait or the disorder is located on the X chromosome. Females have two X chromosomes; males have one X and one Y. Genes on the X chromosome can be recessive or dominant. X-linked recessive genes are expressed in females only if there are two copies of the gene (one on each X chromosome). However, for males, there needs to be only one copy of an X-linked recessive gene in order for the trait or disorder to be expressed. For example, a woman can carry a recessive gene on one of the X chromosomes unknowingly, and pass it on to a son, who will express the trait.

There is a 50 percent chance that daughters carry the gene and can pass it to the next generation. There is a 50 percent chance that a daughter will not carry the gene and, therefore, cannot pass it on. There is a 50 percent chance that sons do not have the gene and will be healthy. However, there is a 50 percent chance that a son will have inherited the gene and will express the trait or disorder.

Hemophilia and Genetics

Hemophilia is an inherited genetic condition, meaning it is passed down through families. It is caused by a defect in the gene that determines how the body makes factors VIII, IX, or XI. These genes are located on the X chromosome, making hemophilia an X-linked recessive disease. Each person inherits two sex chromosomes from their parents. Females have two X chromosomes. Males have one X and one Y chromosome (Fig. 3.7).

Males inherit an X chromosome from their mother and a Y chromosome from their father. Females receive an X chromosome from each parent. Because the genetic defect that causes hemophilia is located on the X chromosome, fathers cannot pass the disease to their sons. This also means that if a male gets the X chromosome with the altered gene from his mother, he'll have hemophilia. A female with one X chromosome that has the altered gene has a 50 percent chance of passing that gene to her children, male or female.

A female who has the altered gene on one of her X chromosomes is typically called a "carrier." This means she may pass the disease to her children but she does not have the disease herself. This is because she has sufficient clotting factors

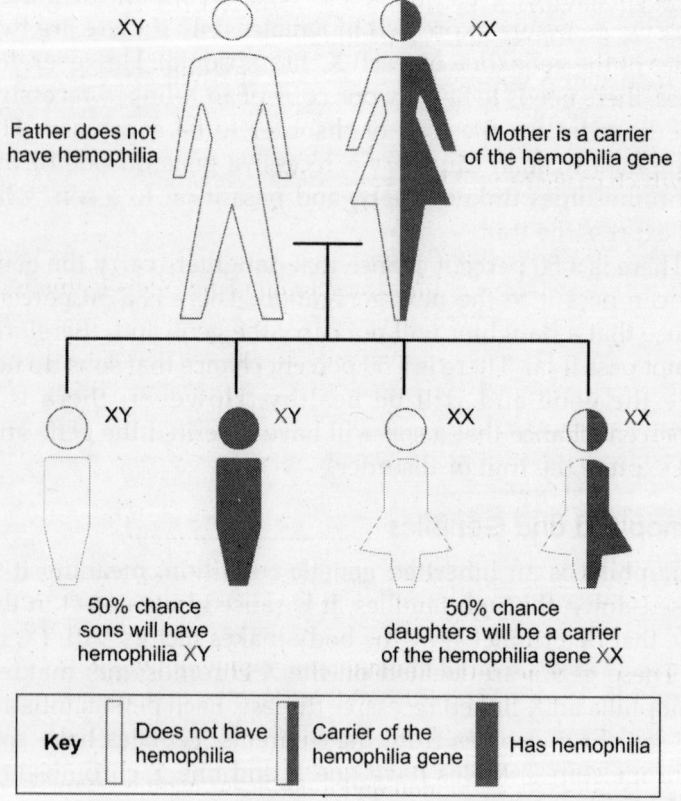

Fig. 3.7: Hemophilia and its inheritance chances

from her normal X chromosome to avoid serious bleeding issues. However, females who are carriers often have an increased risk of bleeding (Queen Victoria was a carrier of hemophilia).

Color Blindness

A normal X chromosome is shown as (X) while a color blind carrying X chromosome is shown in bold (**X**).

The color blind 'gene' is carried on one of the X chromosomes. Since men have only one X chromosome, if his

X chromosome carries the color blind 'gene' (**X**), he will be color blind (**X**Y). A woman can have either:

1. Two normal X chromosomes, so that she will not be color blind or be a carrier (XX),

2. One normal X and one color blind carrying **X** chromosome, in which case she will be a carrier (X**X**), or rarely

3. She will inherit a color blind **X** from her father and a color blind **X** from her mother and be color blind herself (**XX**). She will pass on color blindness to all of her sons if this is the case.

Figures 3.8 to 3.11 show how people can become color blind and how color blindness is passed on to future generations.

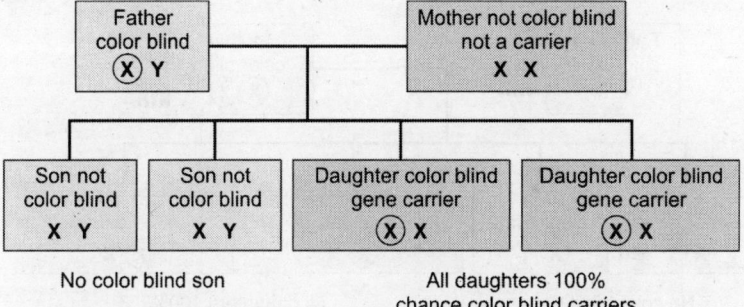

Fig. 3.8: A color blind man and a non-color blind woman

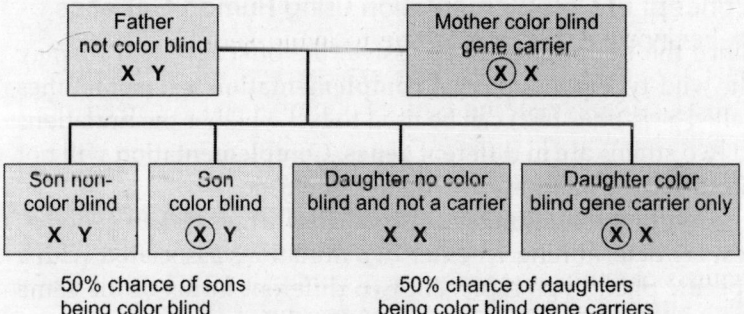

Fig. 3.9: A non-color blind man and a color blind carrier woman

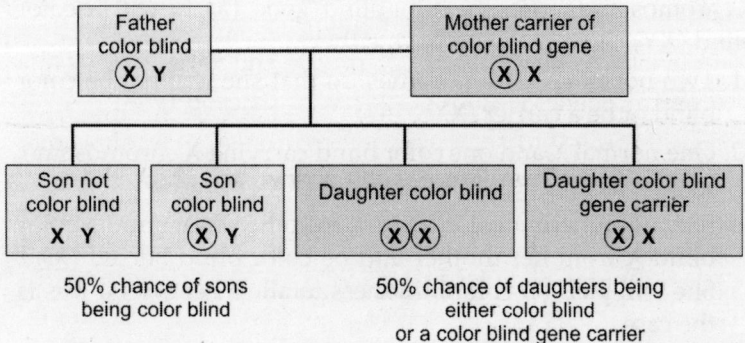

Fig. 3.10: A color blind man and a color blind carrier woman

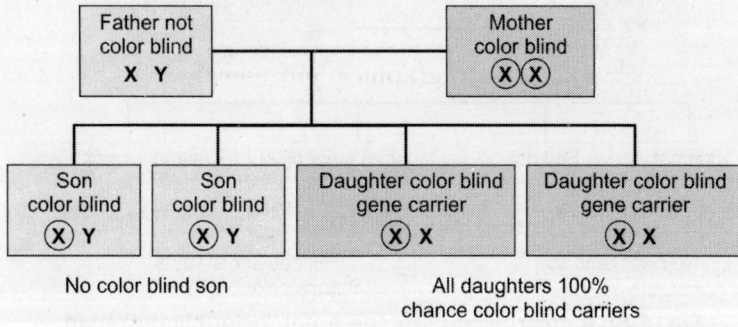

Fig. 3.11: A non-color blind man and a color blind woman

Concept of Complementation Using Human Genetics

Since the mutations are recessive, the offspring will display the wild-type phenotype. A **complementation test** (sometimes called a *cis-trans* test) can be used to **test** whether the mutations in two strains are in different **genes**. **Complementation** will not occur if the mutations are in the same gene.

Complementation test, also called *cis-trans* **test**, in genetics, **test** for determining whether two mutations associated with a specific phenotype represent two different forms of the same gene (alleles) or are variations of two different genes.

KEY POINTS

- Genetics is the study of inheritance and variation.
- Term genetics was first used by W. Bateson 1905.
- Gregor Johann Mendel is called the father of genetics
- Heredity or inheritance is the process by which characters are passed on from parent to progeny.
- Phenotype—external appearance or trait of an individual
- Genotype—genetic constitution of an organism
- Hybrid—the heterozygous organism produced after crossing of genetically different individuals is called hybrid
- Homozygous—both alleles are same/similar for a character, e.g. TT = tall, tt = dwarf.
- Genome—is a complete set of chromosomes where every gene and chromosome is represented singly as in a gamete.
- Punnett square—is a graphical representation to calculate the probability of all genotypes of off springs in a genetic cross—introduced by RC Punnett.
- Genetics is a branch of biology concerned with the study of genes, genetic variation, and heredity in living organisms.
- Gregor Johann Mendel conducted hybridisation experiments on garden pea (*Pisum sativum*) for seven years (1856–1863) and proposed the laws of inheritance in living organisms. He is also known as the Father of Genetics.
- Mendel's laws of inheritance are based on his observations on monohybrid crosses.
- The principle of dominance states that when two alternative forms of a trait or character (genes) are present in an organism, only one factor expresses itself in F1-progeny and is called dominant, while the other that remains masked is called recessive.
- Law of Segregation (First Law)—states that the alleles do not show any blending and both the characters are recovered as such in the F2-generation, though one of these is not seen in the F1-generation.

- Law of Independent Assortment (Second Law) states that when two pairs of traits are combined in a hybrid, segregation of one pair of character is independent of the other pair of characters at the time of gamete formation.
- An allele is an alternative form of a gene (one member of a pair) that is located at a specific position on a specific chromosome.
- The dominant allele is expressed and the recessive allele is masked.
- Multiple alleles: While most genes exist in two allele forms, some have multiple alleles for a trait. Example is ABO blood type.
- **Gene Mapping:** Also called linkage mapping—can offer firm evidence that a disease transmitted from parent to child is linked to one or more genes.
- Genetic Markers: Consist of DNA that does not contain a gene.
- **Gene interaction:** The phenomenon of two or more genes affecting the expression of each other in various ways in the development of a single character of an organism is known as gene interaction.
- Incomplete dominance is a form of intermediate inheritance in which one allele for a specific trait is not completely expressed over its paired allele.
- **Epistasis:** Suppression of the effect of a gene by another gene. One gene completely masks another gene.
- Cells divide and reproduce in two ways—mitosis and meiosis.
- **Mitosis** is a process of cell division that results in two genetically identical daughter cells developing from a single parent cell.
- **Meiosis** is the division of a germ cell involving two fissions of the nucleus and giving rise to four gametes, or sex cells, each possessing half the number of chromosomes of the original cell
- Chromosomes, found in the *cell nucleus*, contain many genes.

- A gene is a section of *DNA*, which carries coding for a particular *protein*. The gene that trumps over the other is usually known as the **dominant gene**, and the weaker gene is known as **recessive**. In the presence of a dominant gene, a recessive gene will not show its traits.

- Single gene disorders are caused by DNA changes in one particular gene

- Albinism caused by lack of pigment melanin in skin, hair and iris of eye.

- Sickle cell anemia—autosomal recessive disease so it is transmitted from parents to offspring when both parents are carrier (heterozygote) for the gene. The disease is controlled by single pair of allels Hb^A and Hb^S.

- **Thalassemia:** It is autosomal recessive disease. It is caused by defect in synthesis of globin polypeptide in RBC resulting in severe anemia.

- X-linked inheritance means that the gene causing the trait or the disorder is located on the X chromosome.

- Hemophilia is an inherited genetic condition caused by a defect factors VIII, IX, or XI genes are located on the X chromosome—X-linked recessive disease.

- The color blind 'gene' is carried on one of the X chromosomes. Since men have only one X chromosome-carries the color blind 'gene'. Women (**XX**) will be color blind.

- **Complementation test**, also called *cis-trans* **test**, in genetics, **test** for determining whether two mutations associated with a specific phenotype represent two different forms of the same gene (alleles) or are variations of two different genes.

PRACTICE QUESTIONS

Very Short Answer Type Questions

1. Who is the father of genetics?
2. Which is dominant gene, round seeds or wrinkled seeds?
3. What is Mendel mono-hybrid ratio?

4. Write down Mendel's dihybrid ratio for phenotypes.
5. What is the location of the gene for hemophilia?
6. What are genotypes of man with blood group A?
7. Mention any 2 of the 7 contrasting traits in garden peas.

Short Answer Type Questions

1. What is genetics?
2. On which plant did Mendel work?
3. What is genotype?
4. What is phenotype?
5. What is dominance?
6. Why did Mendel choose pea plant for his experiments?
7. Differentiate between mono-hybrid and di-hybrid.
8. Differentiate between homozygous and heterozygous.
9. What are multiple alleles?
10. What is epistasis?

Long Answer Type Questions

1. Explain Mendel's law of segregation. Give an example.
2. Explain law of independent assortment.
3. Explain about hereditary diseases with examples.
4. What is gene mapping?
5. Explain how color blindness is passed in children.
6. How genetic material passes from parents to offsprings.
7. Explain the concept of complementation.
8. Explain complementary gene interaction.
9. Explain supplementary gene interaction. Explain the concept of incomplete dominance.

Chapter 4

Biomolecules

SYNOPSIS

This chapter will cover the following topics
1. Introduction to Biomolecules
2. Discussion about monomeric units and polymeric structures
3. Discuss about sugars, starch and cellulose, Amino acids and proteins
4. Discuss about Nucleotides DNA/RNA
5. Discussion about two carbon units and lipids

INTRODUCTION OF BIOMOLECULES

Carbon is the key element of organic compounds. All organic compounds contain carbon. In organic compounds main bond formation takes place between carbon to carbon and carbon to hydrogen. These organic compounds containing carbon, hydrogen and oxygen form the bulk of living organisms. All the carbon compounds from living tissue are the 'biomolecules'.

When various biomolecules or organic substances found in living matter are mixed with tri-chloro acetic acid (Cl_3CCOOH), then two fractions are given out. One fraction which is acid soluble pool forms the filterate and the other fraction which is the acid insoluble pool forms the retentate.

The acid soluble filterate contains chemicals and show a molecular mass of 18 to 800 daltons which are called bio micromolecules. These include amino acids, sugar and nucleotides. Acid insoluble retentate have proteins, nucleic acids, polysaccharides and lipids. All these elements except lipids have a high molecular weight of about 1000 daltons so they are called biomacromolecules. Molecular weight of lipids is not greater than 800 dalton but they come under the acid insoluble retentate as lipids on grinding from vesicles which are not water soluble so lipid fragments in the form of vesicles get separated along with acid insoluble filterate. An organic compound normally present as an essential component of living organism (Fig. 4.1).

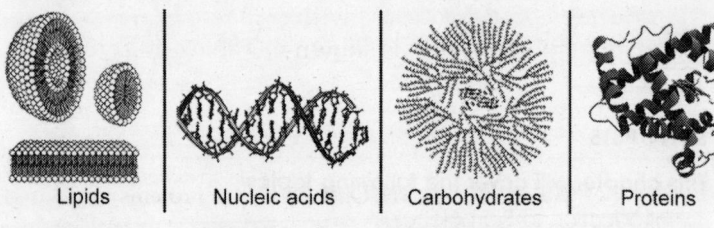

| Lipids | Nucleic acids | Carbohydrates | Proteins |

Fig. 4.1: Biomolecules of life

CHARACTERISTICS OF BIOMOLECULES

1. Most of them are organic compounds.
2. They have specific shapes and dimensions.
3. Functional group determines their chemical properties.
4. Many of them are asymmetric.
5. Macromolecules are large molecules and are constructed from small building block molecules.
6. Building block molecules have simple structure.
7. Biomolecules first gorse by chemical evolution.

IMPORTANT BIOMOLECULES OF LIFE

1. **Water:** Being the universal solvent and major constituents (60%) of any living body without which life is impossible. It acts as a media for the physiological and biochemical reactions in the body itself. Maintain the body in the required turgid condition.
2. **Carbohydrates:** It is very important for source of energy for any physical body function.
3. **Proteins:** These are very important from body maintenance point of view, helps in tissue, cell formation.

4. **Lipids:** These are very important from energy source as well as human nutrition point of view.

5. **Nucleic acids:** Nucleic acids are very important as DNA carries the hereditary information and RNA helps in protein formation for the body.

6. **Enzymes:** Enzymes are simple or combined proteins acting as specific catalysts and activates the various biochemical and metabolic processes within the body. A list of fundamental biomolecules is shown in Table 4.1.

Table 4.1 List of fundamental biomolecules

Sr. No.	Small molecule	Atomic constituents	Derived macro molecule
1	Amino acid	C, H, O, N (S)	Proteins
2	Sugars	C, H, O	Starch, glycogen
3	Fatty acids	C, H, O	Fats, oils
4	Purines and pyrimidine	C, H, O, N	Nucleic acids
5	Nucleotide	C, H, O, N, P	Nucleic acids (DNA and RNA)

Biomolecules is the molecules of life. Four main classes of biomolecules: Carbohydrates, lipids, proteins and nucleic acids. Carbohydrates, proteins and lipids are huge and therefore called macromolecules. Macromolecules are polymers, built from monomers.

1. A polymer is a long molecule consists of many repeating units of monomers as their building blocks.

2. A monomer is a small molecule.

Carbohydrates

Carbohydrates are among the most widely distributed compounds in both plants and animals. Carbohydrates 'hydrates of carbon' are compound mainly made up of carbon, hydrogen and oxygen and are also called saccharides as they are formed of sugars. Carbohydrates are classified as monosaccharides, derived monosaccharides, oligosaccharides and polysaccharides.

Monosaccharides

These sugars are the simple carbohydrates which cannot be hydrolysed further and are made up of 3–7 carbon atoms. Examples are glucose, fructose, galactose, etc

Monosaccharides are generally polyhydroxy aldehydes or ketones. They are named according to number of carbon atoms in the molecule and have the ending '–ose', e.g. triose (3 carbon atoms), tetrose (4 carbon atoms), pentose (5 carbon atoms), hexose (6 carbon atoms), heptose (7 carbon atoms).

OPTICAL ISOMERISM

Many sugars bend the plane of polarized light and exhibit optical isomerism due to presence of asymmetrical carbon atom. A carbon atom is asymmetrical when it has four different groups attached to it.

Glyceraldehyde has one asymmetric carbon and has two optical isomers, dextro rotatory and laevo rotatory form. Dextro rotatory compounds can rotate beam of polarized light to right side and are said as (d) or (+)

Laevo rotatory compounds rotate the plane of polarized light towards left and are labeled (l) or (–) (Fig. 4.2).

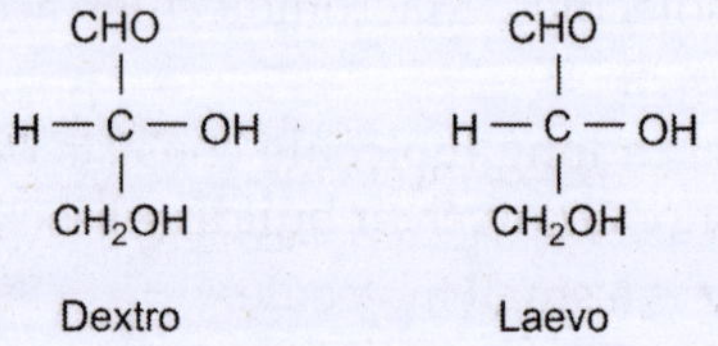

```
        CHO                    CHO
         |                      |
   H — C — OH            H — C — OH
         |                      |
       CH2OH                  CH2OH

       Dextro                 Laevo
```

Fig. 4.2: D and L glyceraldehydes showing optical isomerism

Glucose

Glucose is the most widely distributed sugar. It is sweet tasting and oxidation of glucose provides immediate energy for the cell. Glucose can exist in two forms: Open chain form and the ring form: Open chain form is folded because of tetrahedral bond angles of carbon atom because of this folding, ends of molecule approach each other if carbon atom of aldehyde group is linked to the fifth carbon atom of the chain through an oxygen atom, a ring structure will occur (Fig. 4.3).

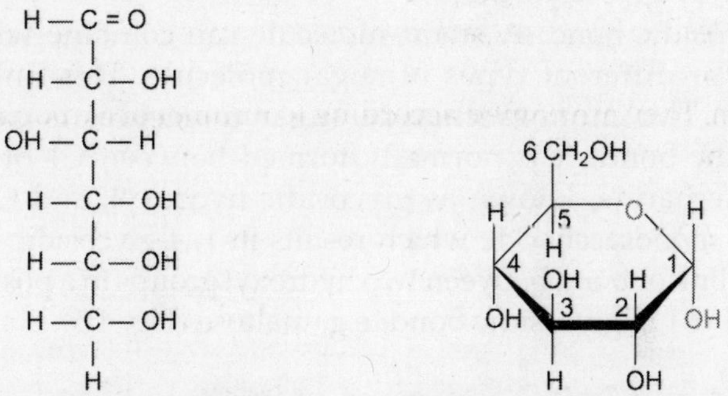

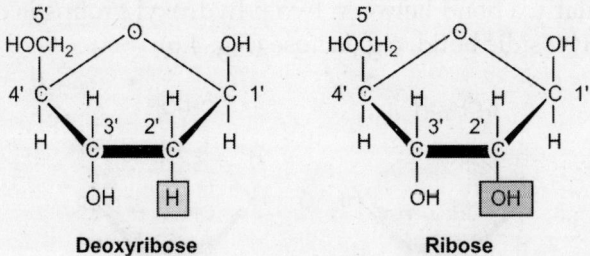

Glucose (straight/ open chain)   Six membering (pyranose) of α glucose

Fig. 4.3: Structure of glucose and pyranose

Derived Monosaccharides

Monosaccharides are modified to form different structures.

Example 1: Deoxy sugar, e.g. deoxygenation which means the removal of oxygen at second carbon of ribose produces deoxyribose (Fig. 4.4).

Deoxyribose   **Ribose**

Fig. 4.4: Modified monosaccharides deoxyribose and ribose

Example 2: Gluconic acid and glucuronic acid. Oxidation of C_1 of glucose to a carboxyl group gives gluconic acids, whereas at C_6 it gives glucuronic acid.

Oligosaccharides

They are small carbohydrates which are formed by condensation (a chemical reaction between two molecules to form one molecule with loss of water molecule) of 2–9 monosaccharides and are biomacromolecules. These monosaccharides are joined together by glycosidic bond.

Glycosidic bond: A sugar molecule can combine with a similar or different types of sugar molecule. This linking between two monosaccharide sugar molecules is called glycosidic bond. It is normally formed between C1 of one monosaccharide, known as glycosidic hydroxyl, and C4 of another monosaccharide which results in 1, 4 glycosidic link. The 1, 4 link or bond between two hydroxyl groups in a position is called α-1, 4 glycosidic bond, e.g. maltose (Fig. 4.5).

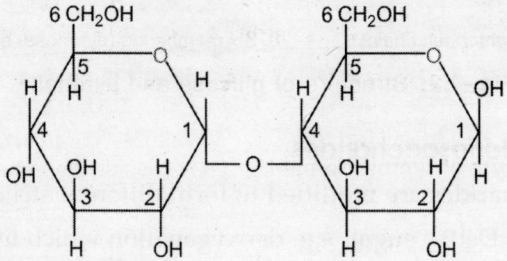

Fig. 4.5: Structure of maltose formed by glycosidic bond between two α-glucose molecule

Similarly a bond between two β-hydroxyl groups is called β-1, 4 glycosidic bond, e.g. lactose (Fig. 4.6).

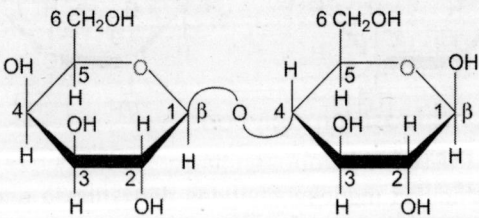

Fig. 4.6: Structure of lactose formed by β-1, 4 glycosidic bond between β-galactose and β-glucose

Glycosidic bond can also form between C1 of one monosaccharide and C6 of another monosaccharide, these bonds occur at point of branching of chain and are called 1, 6 glycosidic bond.

Oligosaccharides are named according to the number of monosaccharide units, i.e. disaccharide contains two monosaccharide units, trisaccharide three, tetrasaccharides four. Disaccharides are the most important of oligosaccharides and occur in both plant and animal cells. A disaccharide is formed by the condensation of two monomers of monosaccharides with removal of water molecule. The important disaccharides are lactose, maltose and sucrose (Fig. 4.7).

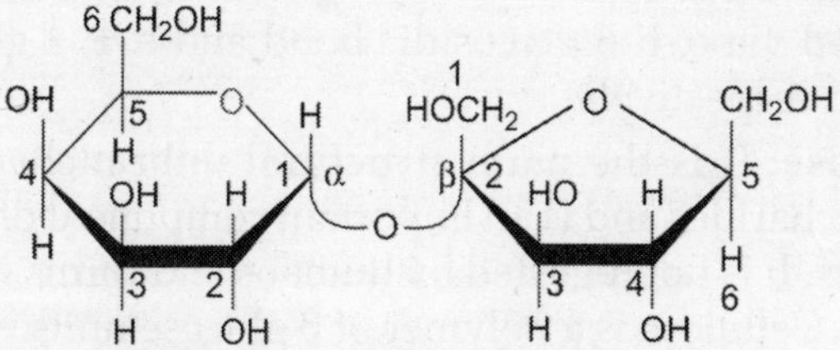

Fig. 4.7: Structure of sucrose formed by 1,6 glycosidic bond between two glucose molecules

Polysaccharides

Polysaccharides are polymers containing at least ten mono-saccharide units and are macromolecules. Polysaccharides contain monosaccharides as building blocks and may be branched or unbranched, these individual monosaccharides are linked by glycosidic bond depending upon their composition. Polysaccharides can be of two kinds: Homopolysaccharides and heteropolysaccharides.

Homopolysaccharides/Homoglycans

Consist of only one type of monosaccharide. Some better known examples of homoglycans are:

1. **Glycogen:** It is made up of 30,000 glucose residues and is the major reserve of carbohydrates in animals and is also called as animal starch. It is stored mainly in liver and muscles. It is an unbranched structure having α-1, 4 linkage at unbranched part and branching parts have α-1, 6 linkage. Glycogen is non-reducing and gives a red color with iodine.

2. **Starch:** It is the carbohydrate reserve in plant cells. Starch is a polymer of α-D-glucose units. Starch has two components.

   i. *Amylase:* It consists of about 200–500 glucose units which are found in a straight chain and consists of α-1, 4 glycosidic linkage between D glucose molecules. It is helical, each turn consists of 6 glucose units. Amylase gives blue color with iodine.

   ii. *Amylopectin:* It consists of 1,000 glucose units and has branched and unbranched glucose units which are linked via α-1, 6 glycosidic bond and α-1, 4 glucosidic bond respectively.

3. **Cellulose:** It is the main structural unbranched homopolysaccharides and is an important component of cell wall of plants. It is not digested by humans and forms roughage of food. Cellulose is a polymer of β glucose units which are joined by β-1, 4 glucosidic bonds. Cotton fibers contain largest (90%) of cellulose wood contains 25–50% cellulose.

4. **Chitin:** It is the second most abundant organic substance and is found in hard endoskeleton of insects. In chitin the basic unit is nitrogen containing glucose derivative called N-acetyl glucosamine.

5. **Inulin:** It is the polymer of fructose. It is found in roots of dahalia inulin is not metabolized in human body and filters out through kidney, so it is used as test for kidney function.

Heteropolysaccharides

Which consist of more than one type of monosaccharides so these can be said as heteropolymer or heteroglycans. Some examples of heteroglycans are:

1. **Peptidoglycan:** It is present in bacterial cell wall. In peptidoglycan heteropolysaccharide chains are made up of alternate amino sugar molecules that is N-acetyl glucosamine and N-acetyl muranmic acid.

2. **Hyaluronic acid:** It acts as a cementing substance in connective tissue and is found in skin, umbilical cord, and vitreous humour of eye. It is a heteropolysaccharide

composed of D-N-acetyl glucosamine and D glucouronic acid.

3. **Chondroitin sulfate:** It is found in cartilage, tendons, skin and saliva. It is a heteropolymer consisting of N-acetyl galactosamine and glucouronic acid.

4. **Pectin** are found in cell wall of plants where it binds cellulose fibrils in bundles. It is composed of methylated galacturonic acid with galactose and arabinose.

AMINO ACIDS

Amino acids are a crucial, yet basic unit of protein, and they contain an amino group and a carboxylic group. They play an extensive role in gene expression processes, which includes the adjustment of protein functions that facilitate messenger RNA (mRNA) translation. In nature, over 700 types of amino acids have been uncovered. Almost all of them are α-amino acids. They have been discovered in: Bacteria; fungi; algae; various other plants. Amino acids are classified as:

1. Nonessential
2. Essential
3. Conditionally essential

The classification as essential or nonessential does not actually reflect their importance, as all 20 amino acids are necessary for human health.

Essential Amino Acids

Eight of these amino acids are essential and cannot be produced by the body, they are:

1. Leucine
2. Isoleucine
3. Lysine
4. Threonine
5. Methionine
6. Phenylalanine
7. Valine
8. Tryptophan

Histidine is an amino acid that is categorized as semi-essential since the human body does not always need it to properly function; therefore, dietary sources of it are not always essential. The conditionally essential amino acids are not usually required in the human diet, but do become essential under certain circumstances.

Nonessential Amino Acids

Nonessential amino acids are produced by the human body either from essential amino acids or from normal protein breakdowns. Nonessential amino acids include

1. Asparagine
2. Alanine
3. Arginine
4. Aspartic acid
5. Cysteine
6. Glutamic acid
7. Glutamine
8. Proline
9. Glycine
10. Tyrosine
11. Serine

An **additional amino acids' classification** depends upon the side chain structure, and experts recognize these five as:

1. Cysteine and Methionine (amino acids containing sulfur)
2. Asparagine, Serine, Threonine, and Glutamine (neutral amino acids)
3. Glutamic acid and Aspartic acid (acidic); and Arginine and Lysine (basic)
4. Leucine, Isoleucine, Glycine, Valine, and Alanine (aliphatic amino acids)
5. Phenylalanine, Tryptophan, and Tyrosine (aromatic amino acids)

One **final amino acid classification** is categorized by the side chain structure that divides the list of 20 amino acids into four groups—two of which are the main groups and two that are subgroups. They are:

1. Non-polar
2. Polar
3. Acidic and polar
4. Basic and polar

For example, side chains having pure hydrocarbon alkyl or aromatic groups are considered non-polar, and these amino acids are comprised of phenylalanine, glycine, valine, leucine, alanine, isoleucine, proline, methionine, and tryptophan. Meanwhile, if the side chain contains different polar groups like amides, acids, and alcohols, they are classified as polar. Their list includes tyrosine, serine, asparagine, threonine, glutamine, and cysteine. If the side chain contains a carboxylic acid, the amino acids in the acidic-polar classification are aspartic acid and glutamic acid. Furthermore, if the side chain consists of a carboxylic acid and basic-polar, these amino acids are lysine, arginine, and histidine (Fig. 4.8).

Properties of Amino Acids

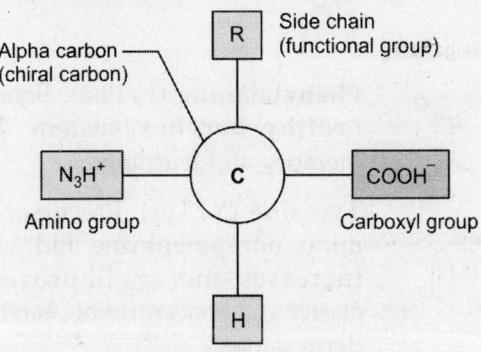

Fig. 4.8: Properties of amino acids

Amino Acids and their Functions

Non-polar aliphatic residues glycine (G/Gly). Slices DNA in order to produce different amino acids. One of the three most important glycogenic amino acids.

Alanine (A/Ala). Important source of energy for muscle. One of the three most important glycogenic amino acids. The primary amino acid in sugar metabolism. Boosts immune system by producing antibodies.

Valine (V/Val). Essential for muscle development.

Leucine (L/Leu). Beneficial for skin, bone and tissue wound healing.

Isoleucine (I/Ile). Necessary for the synthesis of hemoglobin.

Proline (P/Pro). Critical component of cartilage; aids in joint health, tendons and ligaments. Keeps heart muscle strong.

Aromatic Residues

Phenylalanine (F/Phe). Beneficial for healthy nervous system. It boosts memory and learning.

Tyrosine (Y/Tyr). Precursor of dopamine, norepinephrine and adrenaline. Increases energy, improves mental clarity and concentration, can treat some depressions.

Tryptophan (W/Trp). Necessary for neurotransmitter serotonin (synthesis). Effective sleep aid, due to conversion to serotonin. Reduces anxiety and some forms of depression. Treats migraine headaches. Stimulates growth hormone.

Polar Non-charged Residue

Serine (S/Ser). One of the three most important glycogenic amino acids, the others being alanine and glycine. Maintains blood sugar levels, and boosts immune system. Myelin sheaths contain serine.

Threonine (T/Thr). Required for formation of collagen. Helps prevent fatty deposits in liver. Aids in antibodies' production.

Cysteine (C/Cys). Protective against radiation, pollution, and ultra-violet light. Detoxifier; necessary for growth and repair of skin.

Methionine (M/Met). An antioxidant. Helps in breakdown of fats and aids in reducing muscle degeneration.

Asparagine (N/Asn). One of the two main excitatory neurotransmitters.

Glutamine (Q/Gln). Essential for helping to maintain normal and steady blood sugar levels. Helps muscle strength and endurance. Gastrointestinal function; provides energy to small intestines.

Positively Charged Residues

Lysine (L/Lys). Component of muscle protein, and is needed in the synthesis of enzymes and hormones. It is also a precursor for L-carathine, which is essential for healthy nervous system function.

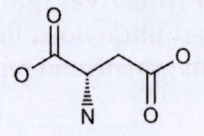

Arginine (R/Arg). One of the two main excitatory neurotransmitters. May increase endurance and decrease fatigue. Detoxifies harmful chemicals. Involved in DNA synthesis.

Histidine (H/His). Found in high concentrations in hemoglobin. Treats anemia; has been used to treat rheumatoid arthritis.

Negatively Charged Residues

Aspartate (D/Asp). Increases stamina and helps protect the liver; DNA and RNA metabolism; immune system function.

Glutamate (E/Glu). Neurotransmitter that is involved in DNA synthesis.

Ionization

At pH of about 6.0, the α-carboxyl group of amino acid is negatively charged and α-amino group is positively charged. As amino acid molecule contains both negative (CO $\bar{\text{O}}$) and positive (NH$_3^+$) group there is no net charge. Such ions are called **Zwitterions** or dipolar ions.

The point at which the molecule has equal positive and negative charges, it is called isoelectric point. At this point amino acid does not migrate in an electric field.

If the pH is lowered the –COOH group ceases to be ionized and molecule becomes positively charged but when the pH is raised, NH$_3^+$ group dissociates to lose a proton and it becomes –NH$_2$. The molecule as a whole then becomes negatively charged because of the negative charge on the (CO$\bar{\text{O}}$) group (Fig. 4.9).

$$NH_3^+$$
$$H — C — COOH$$
$$R$$
pH 1

$$NH_3^+$$
$$H — C — COO^-$$
$$R$$
pH 6

$$NH_2^+$$
$$H — C — COO^-$$
$$R$$
pH 11

$$R$$
$$H_3N^+ — CH — COO^- \quad \text{Zwitter ion}$$

Fig. 4.9: Ionization and zwitter ion

PROTEINS

Proteins are large molecules of high molecular weight. These are needed by our cells need to function properly. They consist of amino acids. All proteins are made up of carbon, hydrogen, oxygen and nitrogen, presence of nitrogen distinguishes proteins from carbohydrates and fats. The structure and function of our bodies depend on proteins. The regulation of the body's cells, tissues, and organs cannot happen without them. Muscles, skin, bones, and other parts of the human body contain significant amounts of protein, including enzymes, hormones, and antibodies. Proteins also work as neurotransmitters. Hemoglobin, a carrier of oxygen in the blood, is a protein.

Protein molecules are essential for the functioning of every cell in the body. The body synthesizes some proteins foods we eat.

Proteins are long chains of amino acids that form the basis of all life. They are like machines that make all living things, whether viruses, bacteria, butterflies, jellyfish, plants, or human function.

The human body consists of around 100 trillion cells. Each cell has thousands of different proteins. Together, these cause each cell to do its job. The proteins are like tiny machines inside the cell.

Types of Protein

There are three types of protein foods

Complete proteins: These foods contain all the essential amino acids. They mostly occur in animal foods, such as meat, dairy, and eggs.

Incomplete proteins: These foods contain at least one essential amino acid, so there is a lack of balance in the proteins. Plant foods, such as peas, beans, and grains mostly contain incomplete protein.

Complementary proteins: These refer to two or more foods containing incomplete proteins that people can combine to supply complete protein. Examples include rice and beans or bread with peanut butter.

Peptides: The term peptide is used when the chain contains 2–20 amino acid residues chain containing 20–50 amino acid residue are called polypeptide and compounds containing more than 50 amino acids residue are called proteins (Fig. 4.10).

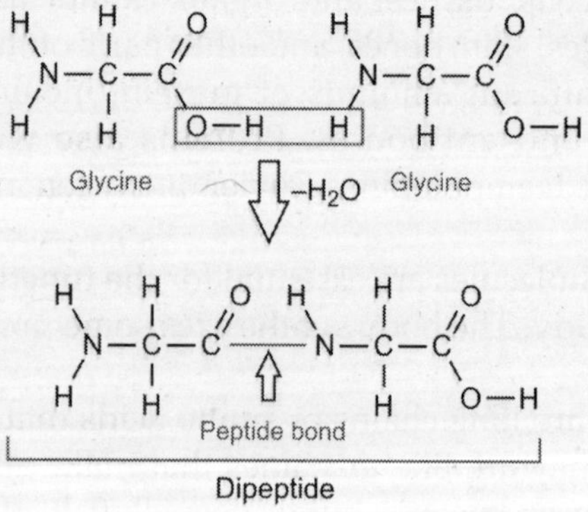

Fig. 4.10: Dipeptide bond

A dipeptide is formed when two amino acids are linked together by a peptide bond with removal of a water molecule. Condensation reaction occurs between ($-NH_2$) group of one amino acid and ($-COOH$) group of another. The dipeptide has an amino group at one end and a carboxyl group at the other.

Classification of Proteins

Proteins may be classified as simple proteins and conjugated proteins.

Simple Proteins

Consists of only amino acid or their derivates. When hydrolysed by acids, alkalies or enzymes simple proteins give only amino acids. These include:

1. **Albumins**—water soluble proteins, e.g. lactalbumin found in milk, serum albumin in blood.
2. **Globulins**—water insoluble, soluble in strong acids/base, e.g. lactoglobulin in milk.
3. **Glutelins**—soluble in dilute acid/alkalies, found in plants.
4. **Histones**—water soluble basic amino acids. These are rich in arginine or lysine. In eukaryotes DNA of chromosomes associate with histones to form nucleoproteins.

Conjugated Protein

It consists of simple proteins in combination with some non protein component. The non-protein part is called prosthetic part. Some examples are:

1. **Nucleoproteins:** These are proteins in combination with nucleic acid like nucleohistones are combination of nucleic acid with protein histones, protamines.
2. **Glycoproteins:** These are proteins in combination with carbohydrate, e.g. immunoglobins secreted by plasma cells, mucin.
3. **Phosphoproteins:** These are proteins in combination with phosphate containing radical, e.g. casein of milk.
4. **Chromoproteins:** These are proteins in combination with pigments, e.g. hemoglobin, hemocyanin (blood of insects)
5. **Lipoproteins:** These are proteins in combination with lipids. These can be: High density lipoproteins (HDL) or low density lipoproteins (LDL), chylomicron.
6. **Metalloproteins:** These are proteins in combination with metals, e.g. ferritin.

Sources

a. Rice and beans together provide complete protein.

b. Protein is one of the essential nutrients, or macronutrients, in the human diet, but not all the protein we eat converts into proteins in our body.

c. When people eat foods that contain amino acids, these amino acids make it possible for the body to create, or synthesize, proteins. If we do not consume some amino acids, we will not synthesize enough proteins for our bodies to function correctly.

d. There are also nine essential amino acids that the human body does not synthesize, so they must come from the diet.

e. Protein provides calories. One gram of protein contains 4 calories. One gram of fat has 9 calories.

NUCLEOTIDES

Definition

A nucleotide is an organic molecule that is the building block of DNA and RNA. Nucleotides are monomers of nucleic acid and are macromolecules. They also have functions related to cell signaling, metabolism, and enzyme reactions. A nucleotide is made up of three parts: a phosphate group, a 5-carbon sugar, and a nitrogenous base. The four nitrogenous bases in DNA are adenine, cytosine, guanine, and thymine. RNA contains uracil, instead of thymine. A nucleotide within a chain makes up the genetic material of all known living things. They also serve a number of functions outside of genetic information storage, as messengers and energy moving molecules.

A series of three nucleotides within the DNA is known as a *codon*, and directs the proteins within the cell to attach a specific protein to a series specified by the rest of the DNA. Special codons even specify to the machinery where to stop and start the process. *DNA translation*, as it is known, converts the information from DNA into the language of proteins. This chain of amino acids can then be properly folded, and provide one of many functions within the cell. Each nucleotide consists of (Fig. 4.11):

1. A phosphate group

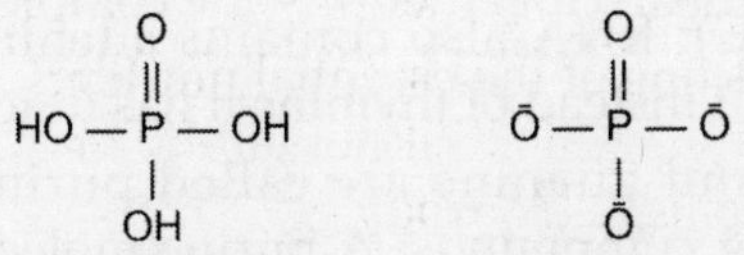

$$
\begin{array}{cc}
\overset{O}{\underset{|}{\overset{||}{HO-P-OH}}} & \overset{O}{\underset{|}{\overset{||}{\bar{O}-P-\bar{O}}}} \\
OH & \bar{O} \\
\text{Phosphoric acid} & \text{Phosphate ion}
\end{array}
$$

Fig. 4.11: Nucleotide showing phosphate group

2. **A five-carbon pentose** sugar deoxyribose which is a pentose sugar with five carbon atoms. Four of the five carbon atoms plus a single oxygen atom form a five membered ring. The fifth carbon atom is outside ring and forms a part of $-CH_2$ group. The four atoms of ring are numbered 1, 2, 3 and 4, whereas carbon atom of $-CH_2$ is numbered 5. Three OH groups are in 1, 3 and 5 positions. Hydrogen atoms are attached to carbon atoms 1, 2, 3 and 4 (Fig. 4.12).

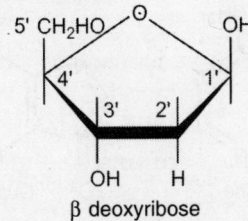

β deoxyribose

Fig. 4.12: Structure of five-carbon pentose sugar deoxyribose

Ribose the pentose sugar of RNA has a similar structure except there is an –OH group attached to H on carbon atom 2 (Fig. 4.13).

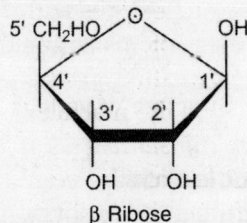

β Ribose

Fig. 4.13: Structure of five-carbon pentose

3. **A heterocyclic nitrogen base:** There are four different bases found in DNA: Adenine (A), guanine (G), thymine (T) and cytosine (C). RNA also contains adenine, guanine and cytosine but instead of thymine it has uracil (U).

Adenine and guanine are called purines. Purines are double ring compounds. A purine molecule consists of a 5-membered imidazole ring attached to a pyrimidine ring.

Cytosine, thymine and uracil are called pyrimidines. Pyrimidines are single ring compounds with nitrogen in positions 1 and 3 (Fig. 4.14).

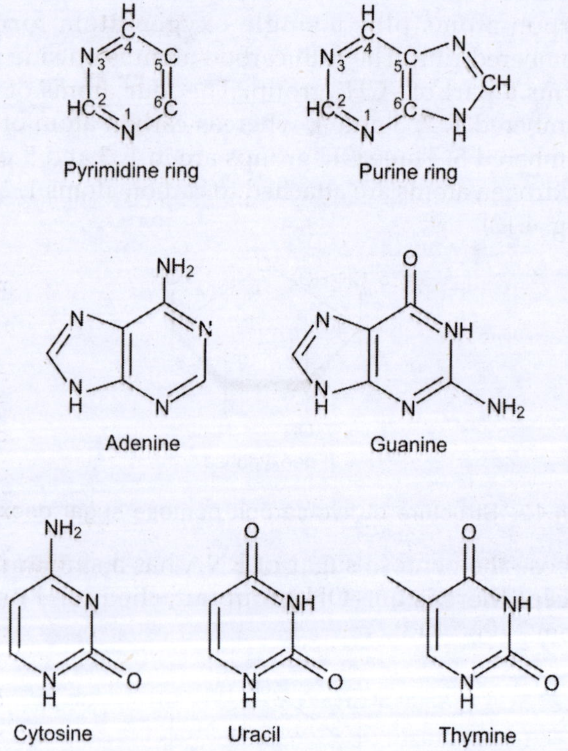

Pyrimidine ring   Purine ring

Adenine   Guanine

Cytosine   Uracil   Thymine

Fig. 4.14: Structure of various nucleotides

Nucleoside and Nucleotide

A sugar molecule and a nitrogenous base forms a nucleoside and a nucleoside plus a phosphate group forms a nucleotide.

Nucleotides of RNA are called ribonucleotides and of DNA are called deoxyribonucleotides. Ribonucleotides contain sugar ribose and deoxyribonucleotides contain the sugar deoxyribose (Fig. 4.15) (Table 4.2).

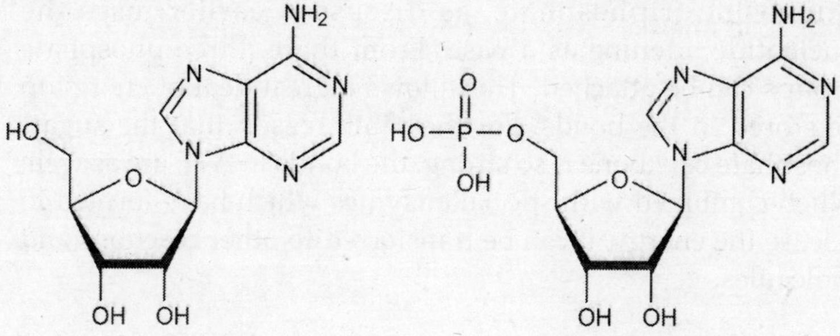

Adenosine (nucleoside)   Adenylic acid (nucleoside)

Fig. 4.15: Structure of various nucleosides

Table 4.2 Various nitrogenous base, nucleoside and nucleotide

	Nitrogenous base	Nucleoside	Nucleotide
1.	Adenine	Adenosine	Adenylic acid
2.	Guanine	Guanosine	Guanylic acid
3.	Cytosine	Cytidine	Cytidylic acid
4.	Thymine	Thymidine	Thymidylic acid
5.	Uracil	Uridine	Uridylic acid

Deoxyribose has two OH groups on carbon 3 and 5 and form nucleotides on 3 and 5 carbon but nucleotides involved in metabolic reactions are generally 5 phosphate esters of nucleoside.

Ribose in a nucleoside has free OH group on carbon 2, 3 and 5 on which phosphate group can attach but most common attachment position of phosphate is at 3 phosphates and 5 phosphates.

Nucleotides involved in metabolic reactions are generally 5 phosphate esters of nucleosides.

Nucleotide Examples

Adenine

Adenine is a purine, which is one of two families of nitrogenous bases. Purines have a double-ringed structure. In DNA, adenine bonds with thymine. In RNA, adenine bonds with uracil. Adenosine triphosphate, as discussed earlier, uses the nucleotide adenine as a base. From there, three phosphate groups can be attached. This allows a great deal of energy to be stored in the bonds. For the same reason that the sugar-phosphate backbone is so strong, the bonds in ATP are as well. When combined with special enzymes which have formed to release the energy, it can be transferred to other reactions and molecules.

Guanine

Like adenine, guanine is a purine nucleotide; it has a double ring. It bonds with cytosine in both DNA and RNA. As seen in the image above, guanine binds to cytosine through three hydrogen bonds. This makes the cytosine-guanine bond slightly stronger than the thymine-adenine bond, which only forms two hydrogen bonds.

Cytosine

Pyrimidines are the other class of nucleotide. Cytosine is a pyrimidine nucleotide; it has only one ring in its structure. Cytosine bonds with guanine in both DNA and RNA. Bonding with the nucleotide guanine, the two make a strong pair.

Thymine

Like the nucleotide cytosine, thymine is a pyrimidine nucleotide and has one ring. It bonds with adenine in DNA. Thymine is not found in RNA. In DNA, it forms only two hydrogen bonds with adenine, making them the weaker pair.

Uracil

Uracil is also a pyrimidine. During transcription from DNA to RNA, uracil is placed everywhere a thymine would normally go. The reason for this is not entirely understood, though uracil has some distinct advantages and disadvantages. Most creatures do not use uracil within the DNA because it is short lived, and can degrade into cytosine. However, in RNA uracil is the preferred nucleotide because RNA is also a short lived molecule.

TYPES OF RIBONUCLEIC ACID (RNA)

Genetic RNA

In the absence of DNA, sometimes RNA functions as genetic material and transfer genetic material from one generation to another, e.g. TMV, QB bacteriophage.

Non-Genetic RNA

These are of three kinds:

1. **Ribosomnal RNA (r-RNA)**
   a. It is the largest RNA and forms 80% of the total RNA.
   b. It is found in ribosomes where protein synthesis takes place.
   c. It is the most stable form of RNA.
   d. There is presence of 80s type of ribosomes in eukaryotes whose subunits are 60s and 40s. In 60s subunit of ribosome – 5s, 5.8s and 28s type of r-RNA can be seen.
   e. In 40s ribosomes 18s r-RNA can be found.
   f. Prokaryotes have 70s type of ribosome which has a subunit of 50s and 30s. In 50s subunit 5s and 23s molecules of r-RNA can be seen, whereas 30s ribosomes has 16 types of r-RNA.

   Function of r-RNA: r-RNA provides attachment site to t-RNA and m-RNA at the time of protein synthesis and attaches them on ribosome.

2. **Transfer RNA (t-RNA) also called soluble or adaptive RNA**
   a. It is the smallest type of RNA and forms 10–15% of total cellular RNA.
   b. It is found in cytoplasm and at the time of protein synthesis it acts as a carrier of amino acids.

  c. The structure of t-RNA is complicated and a scientist Holey gave clover leaf model for its structure in two-dimensional structure but in three-dimensional structure it appears L-shaped.

  d. Function of t-RNA: It acts as a carrier of amino acids at the time of protein synthesis.

3. **Messenger RNA (m-RNA):**

  a. It is produced by genetic DNA in nucleus by a process called transcription.

  b. This m-RNA is 1–5% of the cells total RNA.

  c. m-RNA was discovered by Huxley, Jolkin and Astrachan and the name was given by Jacob and Monad.

Function of m-RNA: m-RNA carries information for protein synthesis.

Functions of Nucleotide

Besides being the basic unit of genetic material for all living things, a nucleotide can have other functions as well. A nucleotide can be a base in another molecule, such as adenosine triphosphate (ATP), which is the main energy molecule of the cell. They are also found in coenzymes like NAD and NADP, which come from ADP; these molecules are used in many chemical reactions that play roles in metabolism. Another molecule that contains a nucleotide is cyclic AMP (cAMP), a messenger molecule that is important in many processes including the regulation of metabolism and transporting chemical signals to cells. Nucleotides not only make up the building blocks of life, but also form many different molecules that function to make life possible.

LIPIDS

A lipid is chemically defined as a substance that is insoluble in water and soluble in alcohol, ether, and chloroform.

Lipids are an important component of living cells. Together with carbohydrates and proteins, lipids are the main constituents of plant and animal cells. Simple lipids include neutral fats and waxes: (1) Neutral fats are also called triglycerides and are the main energy storing compounds in the body. Triglycerides are esters of fatty acid with trihydroxy glycerol when one hydroxyl group of glycerol is esterifies with a fatty acid, a monoglyceride or monoacyl glycerol results.

Fatty Acids

Fatty acid molecule is an unbranched chain of carbon atoms having a carboxylic group attached to an R group. R group can be methyl (CH_3) or ethyl (C_2H_5) or even higher number of carbon group. Fatty acids have the general formula CH_3 $(CH_2)_n COOH$.

The $CH_3 (CH_2)_n CO$—chain is known as acyl radical. Fatty acids vary in chain from acetic acid (C_2) to lignoceric acid (C_{24}). Butyric acid with four carbon atoms is normally the shortest fatty acids found in human fat/the most abundant fatty acids are those having 16 or 18 carbon atoms. For example, palmitic acid has 16 carbons.

The carboxylic acid (–COOH) group of a fatty acid is strongly polar. It ionizes in water at intracellular pH by loss of a proton

$$RCOOH \rightleftharpoons RCO\bar{O} + H^+$$

The hydrocarbon chain is insoluble in water and is nonpolar, so fatty acids have hydrophilic as well as hydrophobic characters.

Fatty acids are divided into

1. **Saturated fatty acids:** Fatty acids which have the maximum possible number of attached hydrogen. Each carbon has two hydrogen atoms attached to it. One of the terminal carbons has three hydrogen atom while other terminal carbon has a carboxyl (COOH) group.

   Example: $CH_3—(CH_2)—COOH$ $\quad$ $CH_3—(CH_2)_{16}—COOH$

   $\quad\quad\quad\quad$ Palmitic acid $\quad\quad\quad\quad\quad\quad$ Stearic acid

2. **Unsaturated fatty acids:** These carbon atoms are not fully saturated with hydrogen and carbon atoms are joined by double bonds removal of hydrogen in stearic acid at carbon 9 and 10 results in the formation of oleic acid which shows double bond between carbon 9 and 10 (Fig. 4.16).

$$CH_3 (CH_2)_7 CH = CH (CH_2)_7 COOH$$

Oleic acid

$$CH_3 (CH_2)_4 CH = CH CH_2 CH = CH (CH_2)_7 COOH$$

Linoleic acid

Fig. 4.16: Unsaturated fatty acids

Cholesterol and triglycerides are lipids. Lipids are easily stored in the body. They serve as a source of fuel and are an important constituent of the structure of cells.

Lipids include fatty acids, neutral fats, waxes and steroids (like cortisone). Compound lipids (lipids complexed with another type of chemical compound) comprise the lipoproteins, glycolipids and phospholipids (Fig. 4.17).

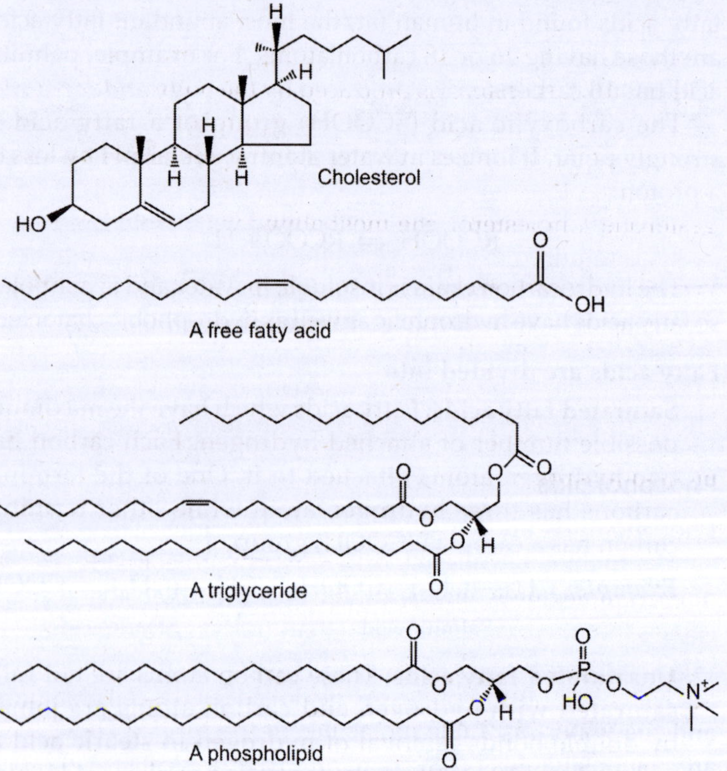

Cholesterol

A free fatty acid

A triglyceride

A phospholipid

Fig. 4.17: Structure of some common lipids

Lipids are fatty, waxlike molecules found in the human body and other organisms. They serve several different roles in the body, including fueling it, storing energy for the future, sending signals through the body and being a constituent of cell membranes, which hold cells together. Lipids are divided into three main types.

Triglycerides

Triglycerides are lipids obtain from food sources of fat, such as cooking oils, butter and animal fat. Triglycerides provide insulation that keeps warm and protects internal organs with a layer of padding. When all the calories are consumed they convert triglycerides for future use.

Steroids

Steroids are a type of lipid that includes hormones and cholesterol. Cholesterol is produced by the body and consumed through food, and it plays a role in the production of hormones. Hormones include the sex hormones estrogen and testosterone, as well as other hormones like adrenaline, cortisol and progesterone. Cholesterol, the most abundant steroid lipid in the body, is required in every cell in the body. It plays a role in cell repair and the formation of new cells. However, too much cholesterol is a bad thing. When it combines with other compounds in blood, it can build up as plaque in arteries, blocking blood flow to and from the heart. Having a high cholesterol level increases the risk of cardiovascular disease

Phospholipids

Phospholipids are derivatives of triglycerides. They are very similar to them but slightly different on a molecular level. Half of each molecule is water-soluble and the other is not, which causes them to react differently than triglycerides. Located on cell membranes, they form double-layered membranes with the water-soluble molecules on the outside of the cell membrane and the water-insoluble molecules in the inside. These lipids are responsible for protecting and insulating cells

Types of Lipids

In the year 1943 Bloor proposed the following classification of lipids based on their chemical composition (Fig. 4.18).

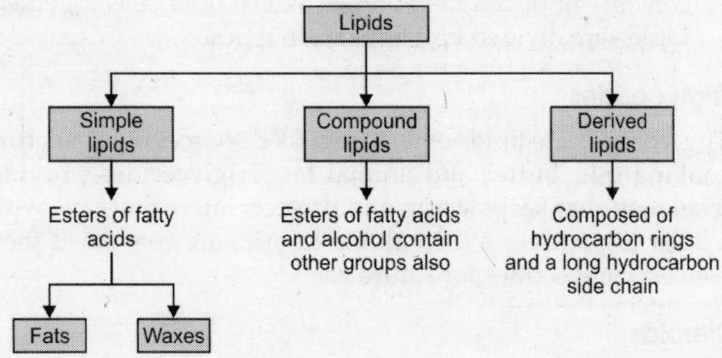

Fig. 4.18: Simple, compound and derived lipids

Simple Lipids

Simple lipids are the esters of fatty acids with various alcohols.

Fats and oils (triglycerides and triacylglycerols): These are esters of fatty acids with a trihydroxy alcohol, glycerol. A fat is solid at ordinary room temperature and oil is liquid.

Simple triglycerides: Simple triglycerides are one in which three fatty acids radicals are of the same type. Example: Tristearin, Triolein.

Mixed triglycerides are one in which the three fatty acids radicals are different from each other. Example: Distearo-olein.

Waxes are the esters of fatty acids with high molecular weight monohydroxy alcohols. Examples: Beeswax, Carnauba wax.

Compound Lipids

They are esters of fatty acids with alcohol and possess additional groups also.

Phospholipids are compound containing fatty acids and glycerol in addition to a phosphoric acid, nitrogen bases and other substituents. They usually possess one hydrophilic head and two non-polar tails.

Phospholipids can be phosphoglycerides, phosphoinositides and phosphosphingosides.

Phosphoglycerides are major phospholipids, they are found in membranes. Examples: Lecithin, Cephalins.

Phosphoinositides are said to occur in phospholipids of brain tissue and soybeans. They play important role in transport processes in cells.

Phosphosphingosides are commonly found in nerve tissue. Example: Sphingomyelins.

Glycolipids are the compounds of fatty acids with carbohydrates and contain nitrogen but no phosphoric acid. The glycolipids also include certain structurally related compounds comprising the groups gangliosides, sulpholipids and sulfatids.

Derived Lipids

Derived lipids are the substances derived from simple and compound lipids by hydrolysis. The most common derived lipids are steroids, terpenes and carotenoids.

Steroids do not contain fatty acids, they are nonsaponifiable, and are not hydrolyzed on heating. They are widely distributed in animals, where they are associated with physiological processes. Example: Estranes.

Terpenes in majority are found in plants. Example: Natural rubber.

Carotenoids are tetraterpenes. They are widely distributed in both plants and animals. They are exclusively of plant origin. Examples: Lycopreene, carotenes, Xanthophylls.

Functions of Lipids

1. Lipids are storage compounds, triglycerides serve as reserve energy of the body.
2. Lipids are important component of cell membranes structure in eukaryotic cells.
3. They act electrical insulators to the nerve fibres, where the myelin sheath contains lipids.

4. Some lipids like prostaglandins and steroid hormones act as cellular metabolic regulators.

5. As lipids are small molecules and are insoluble in water, they act as signalling molecules.

6. Layers of fat in the subcutaneous layer, provides insulation and protection from cold. Body temperature maintenance is done by brown fat.

7. Polyunsaturated phospholipids are important constituents of phospholipids, they provide fluidity and flexibility to the cell membranes.

8. Lipoproteins that are complexes of lipids and proteins, occur in blood as plasma lipoprotein, they enable transport of lipids in aqueous environment, and their transport throughout the body.

9. Essential fatty acids like linoleic and linolenic acids are precursors of many different types of ecosanoids including prostaglandins, thromboxanes. These play a important role in pain, fever, inflammation and blood clotting.

KEY POINTS

- Carbon is the key element of organic compounds.
- Water: Being the universal solvent and major constituents (60%) of any living body.
- Carbohydrates: Important for source of energy for any physical body function.
- Proteins: Important body maintenance point of view, helps in tissue, cell formation.
- Lipids: Important energy source as well as human nutrition point of view.
- Nucleic Acids: Important as DNA carry the hereditary information.
- Enzymes: Simple or combined proteins acting as specific catalysts and activates the various biochemical and metabolic processes within the body.
- Four main classes of biomolecules are carbohydrates, lipids, proteins and nucleic acids.

- Carbohydrates are among the most widely distributed compounds in both plants and animals.
- Carbohydrates 'hydrates of carbon' are compound mainly made up of carbon, hydrogen and oxygen. Carbohydrates are classified as monosaccharides, derived monosaccharides, oligosaccharides and polysaccharides.
- Monosaccharides: Simple carbohydrates which cannot be hydrolysed further and are made up of 3–7 carbon atoms. Examples are glucose, fructose.
- Oligosaccharides: Small carbohydrates which are formed by condensation (a chemical reaction between two molecules to form one molecule with loss of water molecule) of 2–9 monosaccharides and are biomacro-molecules. These monosaccharides are joined together by glycosidic bond.
- Glycosidic bond: A sugar molecule can combine with a similar or different types of sugar molecule.
- Polysaccharides are polymers containing at least ten monosaccharide units and are macromolecules.
- Heteropolysaccharides: Consist of more than one type of monosaccharides so these can be said as heteropolymer or heteroglycans. Examples of heteroglycans are peptidoglycan, hyaluronic acid.
- Amino acids are classified as:
  1. Nonessential
  2. Essential
  3. Conditionally essential
- Essential amino acids: Eight of these amino acids are essential and cannot be produced by the body, they are leucine, isoleucine, lysine, threonine, methionine, phenyl-alanine, valine and tryptophan.
- Nonessential amino acids are produced by the human body either from essential amino acids or from normal protein breakdowns. Example: Asparagine.
- Zwitterions: Amino acid containing both negative ($CO\bar{O}$) and positive (NH_3^+) group, there is no net charge. Such ions are called zwitterions or dipolar ions.

- Isoelectric point: The point at which the molecule has equal positive and negative charges, at this point amino acid does not migrate in an electric field.
- Proteins are large molecules of high molecular weight. These are needed by our cells need to function properly. They consist of amino acids.
- All proteins are made up of carbon, hydrogen, oxygen and nitrogen, presence of nitrogen distinguishes proteins from carbohydrates and fats.
- Protein molecules are essential for the functioning of every cell in the body.
- Types of protein: There are three types of protein foods
  1. *Complete proteins:* These foods contain all the essential amino acids. They mostly occur in animal foods, such as meat, dairy, and eggs.
  2. *Incomplete proteins:* These foods contain at least one essential amino acid, so there is a lack of balance in the proteins. Plant foods, such as peas, beans, and grains, mostly contain incomplete protein.
  3. *Complementary proteins:* These refer to two or more foods containing incomplete proteins that people can combine to supply complete protein. Examples include rice and beans or bread with peanut butter.
- Simple proteins: Consists of only amino acid or their derivates. Example: Albumins.
- Conjugated proteins: Consist of simple proteins in combination with some non-protein component. The non-protein part is called prosthetic parts. Examples: Nucleoproteins, metalloproteins.
- Nucleotide is an organic molecule that is the building block of DNA and RNA.
- A series of three nucleotides within the DNA is known as a *codon.*
- Adenine and guanine are called purines. Purines are double ring compounds. A purine molecule consists of a 5-membered imidazole ring attached to a pyrimidine ring.

- Cytosine, thymine and uracil are called pyrimidines. Pyrimidines are single ring compounds with nitrogen in positions 1 and 3.
- Nucleoside and nucleotide: A sugar molecule and a nitrogenous base forms a nucleoside and a nucleoside plus a phosphate group forms a nucleotide.
- Nucleotides of RNA are called ribonucleotides and of DNA are called deoxyribonucleotides.
- Lipids are chemically defined as a substance that is insoluble in water and soluble in alcohol, ether, and chloroform.
- Lipids are an important component of living cells.
- Phospholipids are derivatives of triglycerides.

PRACTICE QUESTIONS

Very Short Answer Type Questions

1. What are biomolecules?
2. What is the molecular weight of lipids?
3. Give one example of homo-polysaccharides.
4. Which polysaccharide is found in bacterial cell wall?
5. What is chondroitin sulphate made of?
6. What is hyaluronic acid made of?
7. Give one example of conjugated protein?
8. What are the three kinds of RNA?
9. Give one example of steroids.
10. Give the molecular formula of palmitic acid.

Short Answer Type Questions

1. What are carbohydrates?
2. What are dextro-rotatory compounds? Give examples.
3. Draw the structure of glucose.
4. How is maltose formed?
5. What is glycogen?
6. Give differences between (a) essential and non-essential amino acids, (b) saturated and unsaturated fatty acids.

7. What is zwitterion?

8. What are purenes?

9. What are pyrimidines?

10. Give the functions of r-RNA.

Long Answer Type Questions

1. What are oligosaccharides? Explain the formation of lactose.

2. Explain one example of derived mono-saccharide with structure.

3. Explain any two homo-polysaccharides.

4. What are peptides? How is a di-peptide bond formed? Explain with structure.

5. What are nucleotides?

6. Explain the structure of purenes.

7. What are waxes?

8. What are derived lipids?

Enzymes

CATALYSIS

Humans have known about catalysis for many centuries, even though they knew nothing about the chemical process that was involved. The making of soap, the fermentation of wine to vinegar, and the leavening of bread are all processes involving catalysis. In **1812 Russian chemist Gottlieb Sigismund Constantin Kirchhof** studied the behavior of starch in boiling water. Under most circumstances, Kirchhof found, no change occurred when starch was simply boiled in water. But adding just a few drops of concentrated sulfuric acid to the boiling water had a profound effect on the starch. In very little time, the starch broke down to form the simple sugar known as glucose. When Kirchhof found that the sulfuric acid remained unchanged at the completion of the experiment, he concluded that it had simply played a helping role in the conversion of starch to sugar.

Catalysis reactions are usually categorized as either homogeneous or heterogeneous reactions. A homogeneous catalysis reaction is one in which both the catalyst and the substances are in the same phase, i.e either solid, liquid or gas. A heterogeneous catalysis reaction is one in which the catalyst is in a different phase from the substances on which it acts.

Some of the most interesting and important catalysts are those that occur in living systems: The enzymes. All of the reactions that take place within living bodies occur naturally, whether or not a catalyst is present. But they take place so slowly on their own that they are of no value to the survival of an organism. For example, when a sugar cube is placed in a glass of water, it eventually breaks down into simpler molecules with the release of energy. But that process might take years. A person who ate a sugar cube and had to wait that long for the energy to be released in the body would die. Our body also contains catalysts (enzymes) that speed up such reactions. They make it possible for the energy stored in sugar molecules to be released in a matter of minutes.

INTRODUCTION OF ENZYMES

An enzyme is a specialized protein produced with an organism which is capable of catalyzing a specific chemical reaction. Since the enzyme acts as a catalyst, it is also called a biocatalyst. A catalyst influences the rate of a chemical reaction, usually without undergoing any change itself so in this respect an enzyme differs from a normal catalyst.

STRUCTURE OF ENZYMES

All enzymes are proteins which are high molecular weight macromolecules. An enzyme may consist of a single poly-peptide chain or a cluster of polypeptide chains. A polypeptide chain is made up of number of amino acid units linked by peptide bonds.

The sequence and number of the 20 amino acids which make up enzyme varies in different enzymes. This arrangement of enzymes is specific for a particular enzyme and determines the properties of the enzyme. The polypeptide chain has an amino ($-NH_2$) terminal and a carboxyl ($-COOH$) terminal biosynthesis of the enzyme begins at amino terminal.

The different parts of the polypeptide chain are linked by disulphide (-S-S-) bridges. These bridges may be within a polypeptide chain or may connect two polypeptide chains.

ACTIVE SITE

An enzyme has a distinct cavity or cleft in which the substrate is bound. A substrate is a specific compound acted upon by an enzyme. The part of the enzyme where the substrate binds is called the **active site** (since that is where the catalytic "action" happens).

$$\text{For example:} \quad CO_2 \quad + \quad H_2O \longrightarrow H_2CO_3$$
$$\text{Carbon dioxide} \quad \text{Water} \quad \text{Carbonic acid}$$

In the absence of the enzyme carbonic anhydrase this reaction is very slow, producing two hundred molecules of carbonic anhydrase in an hour but in the presence of carbonic anhydrase present in the cytoplasm, this reaction speeds up dramatically with roughly six lakhs molecules formed every second.

NATURE OF ENZYME ACTION

As we already know that an enzyme has a distinct cavity in which substrate bounds. The cleft contains an active centre in which amino acids are grouped together in such a way as to enable them to combine with substrate, it is the chemical which converts into a product. Thus enzymes include active sites which are capable of converting substrate (S) into a product (P).

$$S \longrightarrow P$$
$$\text{(Substrate)} \quad \text{(Product)}$$

1. The substrate 'S' binds to the active site of the enzyme for which it has to diffuse towards the active site. There is the formation of 'ES' (enzyme substrate) complex. This complex formation lasts for a short time and is called transient phenomenon.

2. When substrate binds to the active site of enzyme a new structure of the substrate called transition state structure is formed.

3. The molecules of the substrate group undergo chemical changes, breaking or making of bonds and finally the product is formed and is released from the active site.

4. The pathways of this transformation of substrate into product must go through the so called transition state structure.

5. The molecules of the substrate group undergo chemical changes, breaking or making of bonds and finally the product is formed and is released from the active state.

6. The pathways of this transformation of substrate into product must go through the so called transition structure. There can be many altered structural states between the stable substrate and the product. In this change of substrate to product, all intermediate structural states are unstable.

How do Enzymes Catalyze Reaction

Each enzyme has an active site to which substrate binds and forms a short-lived highly reactive enzyme substrate complex. This is followed by enzyme product complex (EP). Finally the enzyme product complex dissociates into product (P) and the enzyme freed, remains unchanged and is able to bind more substrate molecules (Fig. 5.1).

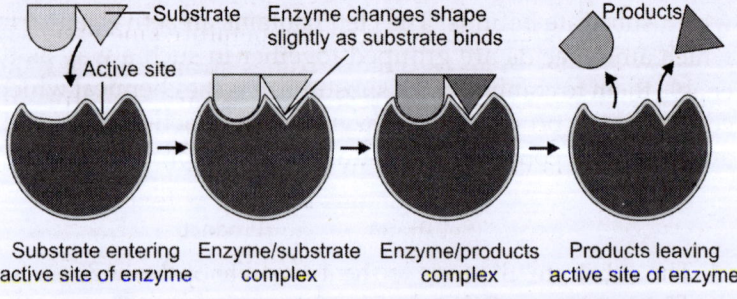

Fig. 5.1: Substrate and active site binding mechanism

The formation of the ES complex is essential for catalysis

$$E + S = ES \rightarrow EP \rightarrow E + P$$

The catalytic cycle of an enzyme can be described as:

1. The substrate binds to the active site of enzyme
2. The binding of the substrate induces the enzyme to alter its shape and fit tightly around the substrate.
3. The active site of the enzyme which is in close proximity of the substrate break the chemical bonds of the substrate and an enzyme product complex is formed.
4. The enzyme releases the products of the reaction and the free enzyme is ready to take up another molecule of substrate.

FACTORS AFFECTING ENZYME ACTIVITY

Enzymes are proteins with tertiary structure. Any change in tertiary structure would affect the action of enzymes. Factors which affect enzyme action are as follows:

1. **Temperature:** Enzyme action is greatly affected by temperature. The temperature at which enzymes show their highest activity is called optimum temperature. Enzyme activity declines both above and below the optimum temperature. At low temperature, enzymes become temporarily inactive and increasing the temperature to normal, they regain their lost activity. At high temperature there is a loss of enzyme activity due to protein denaturation. At higher temperature kinetic energy of molecules in an enzyme becomes strong to break the weak hydrogen bond present in tertiary structure of enzyme resulting in loss of catalytic activity. This change in structure is called denaturation of enzyme. Once an enzyme denatures, it remains inactive as temperature is lowered down (Fig. 5.2).

   The optimum temperature for human enzymes is 35–40°C. The enzyme activity decreases with decrease as well as increase in temperature and stops at 0°C and above 80°C.

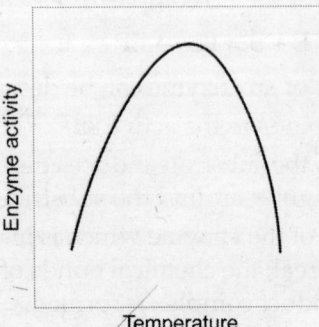

Fig. 5.2: Effect of change in temperature on enzyme activity

2. **pH:** At optimum pH the activity of enzymes is maximum for most enzymes, the effective pH range is 4–9. Beyond these limits denaturation of enzymes takes places. For example, the optimum pH for pepsin is 2 and for trypsin is 8 (Fig. 5.3).

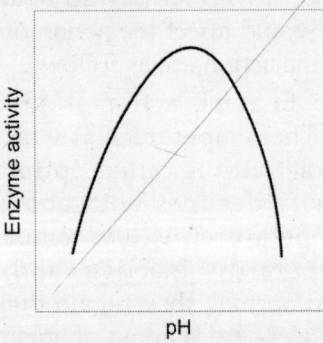

Fig. 5.3: Effect of change in pH on enzyme activity

3. **Concentration of substrate:** Increase in substrate concentration, increases the velocity of enzymatic reaction. The reaction soon reaches a maximum velocity (V_{max}) which is not exceed by further rise in concentration of substrate. This is because, at this stage the enzyme molecules become fully saturated and no active site is left free to bind to additional substrate molecules.

4. **Product concentration:** Accumulation of the product of enzyme reaction lowers the enzyme activity. Enzyme molecules must be freed to combine with more substrate

molecules. Normally the products are quickly removed from the site of formation and reaction does not suffer.

NOMENCLATURE AND CLASSIFICATION OF ENZYMES

Enzymes are generally named by adding 'ase' to the root indicating the substrate on which the enzyme acts. The International Union of Biochemistry report of 1962 contains a scheme for enzyme classification. Enzymes have been divided into 6 groups.

1. **Oxireductases dehydrogenases:** Enzymes which catalyze oxidation reduction reactions involving transfer of electrons/H^+ from one molecule to another, in these reactions one compound is oxidized and the other is reduced.

   Example: Dehydrogenase, oxidase, reductase

   $$\text{Alcohol} + \text{NAD} \longrightarrow \text{Aldehyde} + \text{NADH}_2$$

2. **Transferases:** These enzymes catalyse the transfer of specific group other than hydrogen from one substrate to another.

   Example: Kinase catalyse the phosphorylation of substrate by transferring phosphate group from ATP.

3. **Hydrolysis:** These enzymes catalyze the breakdown of larger molecules into smaller molecules with the addition of water. These bring hydrolysis of ether, peptide and ester.

   Examples: Amylase, lipase, maltase

   $$\text{Sucrose} + \text{H}_2\text{O} \longrightarrow \text{Glucose} + \text{Fructose}$$

4. **Lyases:** These enzymes catalyze the cleavage of substrate into two parts, without the use of water or removal of group without hydrolysis. A double bond is formed at the place of removal of group.

   Examples: Decarboxylase, carbonic anhydrase, etc.

5. **Isomerase:** These enzymes catalyse the rearrangement of molecular structure to form isomers. Isomers are the molecular compounds that are similar in having the same molecular formula but have different arrangement of atoms. Example: Isomerase

   $$\text{Glucose-6-phosphate} \underset{}{\overset{\text{isomerase}}{\rightleftharpoons}} \text{Fructose-6-phosphate}$$

6. **Ligases:** These enzymes catalyse covalent bonding of two substrates to form a large molecule. They catalyze joining of C-O, C-S, P-O bonds by using ATP as energy source.

Examples: RUBP carboxylase, phosphophenol pyruvate (PEP)

$$\begin{matrix} \text{phosphophenol} \\ \text{pyruvic acid} \end{matrix} + CO_2 \xrightarrow[\text{PEP}]{\text{ATP}} \text{ozaloacetic acid}$$

MECHANISM OF ENZYME ACTION

Two hypotheses have been put forward to explain the mode of enzyme action.

1. **Lock and key hypothesis:** This hypothesis was given by Emil Fischer in 1984. According to this hypothesis, both enzyme and substrate molecules have specific geometrical shapes. It is similar to the system of lock and key, which have special geometrical shapes in the region of their activity. The active site contains special groups having $-NH_2$, $-COOH$, $-SH$ for establishing contact with the substrate molecules. Just as a lock can be opened by its specific key, a substrate molecule can be acted upon by a particular enzyme. This explains the specificity of enzyme action. After coming in contact with the active site of enzyme, the substrate molecule forms a complex called enzyme substrate complex. In this enzyme substrate complex, the molecules of the substrate undergo chemical change and form products. The product no longer fits into the active site and escapes in surrounding medium, leaving the active site free to receive more substrates molecules (Fig. 5.4).

Enzyme + Substrate $\longrightarrow$ Enzyme – Substrate Complex

Enzyme – Substrate Complex $\longrightarrow$ Enzyme + End Products

This theory explains how a small concentration of enzyme can act upon a large amount of the substrate. It also explains how the enzyme remains unaffected at the end of chemical reaction. The theory explains how a substance having a structure similar to the substrate can work as a competitive inhibitor.

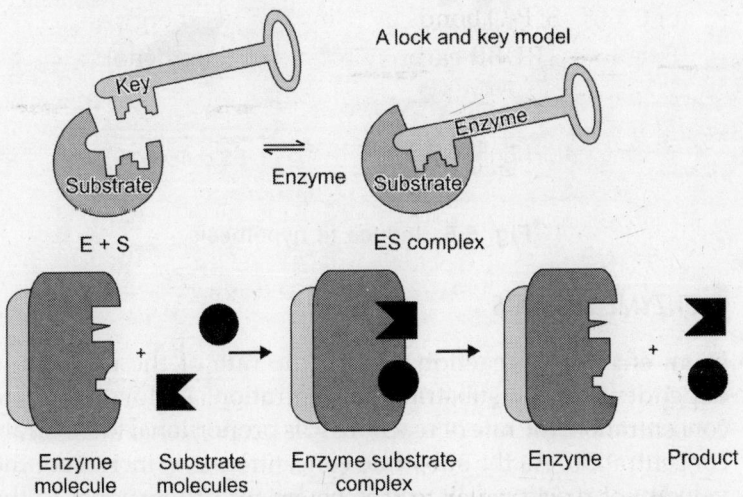

Fig. 5.4: Lock and key hypothesis to show the specificity of enzymes

2. **Induced fit hypothesis:** This hypothesis was proposed by Koshland in 1960. According to this hypothesis, the active site of the enzyme does not initially exist in a shape that is complementary to the substrate but is induced to assume the complementary shape as the substrate becomes bound to the enzyme. According to Koshland, the active site reaches a complementary shape in a similar way as a hand induces a change in the shape of glove. An active site of an enzyme is a crevice or a pocket into which the substrate fits. Thus, enzymes through their active site, catalyze reactions at a higher rate. Hence according to this model, the enzyme and its active site is flexible and the active site of the enzyme contains two groups:

  a. Buttressing group meant for supporting substrate.
  b. Catalytic group meant for catalyzing the reaction when . substrate comes in contact with the buttressing group, the active site changes to bring the catalytic group opposite the substrate bonds to be broken (Fig. 5.5).

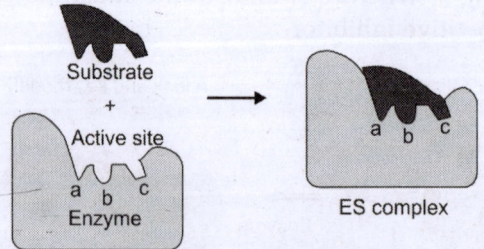

Fig. 5.5: Induce fit hypothesis

ENZYME KINETICS

In an enzymatic reaction S → P, the rate of the reaction is dependent on the substrate concentration. At low substrate concentration, the rate of reaction 'v' is proportional to substrate concentration. As the substrate concentration is increased, the velocity of reaction falls and is no longer proportional to the substrate concentration. With the further increase in substrate concentration, the rate of reaction becomes constant and independent of substrate concentration. The enzyme at this stage shows the saturation effect, i.e. it has become saturated with the substrate and levels off to a flat plateau at high substrate concentration.

The plateau occurs because the enzyme is saturated, meaning all available enzyme molecules are tied up with substrates. Any additional substrate molecule will have to wait around till another enzyme is available, so we can say rate of reaction is limited by enzyme concentration. This maximum rate of reaction is characteristic of a particular enzyme at a particular concentration and is known as the maximum velocity or V_{max}.

The substrate concentration that gives a rate that is halfway to V_{max} is called K_m and is a useful measure of how quickly reaction rate increases with substrate concentration. K_m is also a measure of an enzyme affinity (tendency to bind) to its substrate. A low K_m corresponds to a higher affinity for substrate, while a higher K_m corresponds to a lower affinity for the substrate.

This saturation effect led Michaelis and Menten to a general theory of enzyme action and kinetics in the year 1913 (Fig. 5.6).

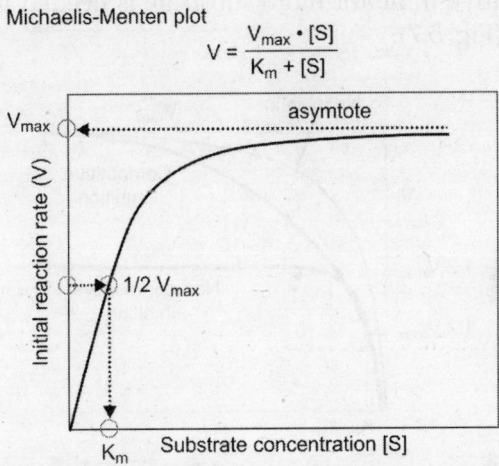

Michaelis-Menten plot

$$V = \frac{V_{max} \cdot [S]}{K_m + [S]}$$

Fig 5.6: Effect of change in concentration of substrate on enzyme activity

$$S = \text{Substrate}$$
$$V = \text{Reaction velocity}$$
$$V_{max} = \text{Maximum velocity}$$
$$K_m = \text{Michaelis-Menten constant}$$

INHIBITION OF ENZYME ACTION

Any substance which can diminish the velocity of an enzyme catalysed reaction is called inhibitor. They act in three different ways.

1. **Competitive inhibition:** This type of inhibition occurs when the inhibitor binds reversibly at the same site where substrate would normally bind and therefore competes with the substrate for that site.

   Effect on V_{max}: The effect of a competitive inhibitor can be reversed by increasing substrate. At a high substrate concentration, the reaction velocity reaches V_{max} as observed in the absence of inhibitor.

Effect on K_m: A competitive inhibitor increases K_m for the given substrate. This means that in the presence of competitive inhibitor more substrate is needed to achieve $\frac{1}{2}\, V_{max}$ (Fig. 5.7).

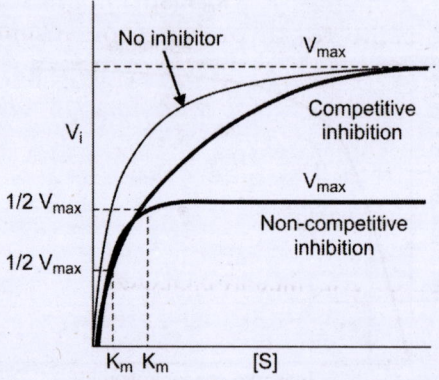

Fig. 5.7: Effect of a competitive inhibitor on the reaction velocity (V_0) versus substrate [S] plot

2. **Non-competitive inhibition:** This inhibition is brought about by a substance which does not resemble the substrate in structure. This non-competitive inhibitor binds to the enzyme at some site other than the substrate binding site, thus no product is formed.

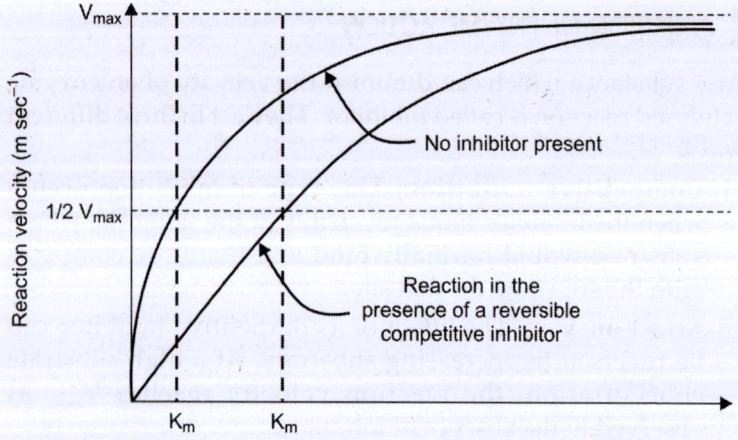

Fig. 5.8: Effect of a non-competitive inhibitor on the reaction velocity (V_0) versus substrate [S] plot

Effect on V_{max}: Non-competitive inhibitor cannot be overcome by increasing the concentration of substrate, so non-competitive inhibitors decrease the V_{max} of the reaction.

Effect on K_m: Non-competitive inhibitors do not interfere with binding of substrate to enzyme. Thus the enzyme shows the same K_m in presence or absence of non-competitive inhibitor.

3. **Allosteric inhibition:** Some inhibitors join an enzyme at a specific site and change the form of the active site meant for the substrate. These inhibitors are also known as modifiers.

IMPORTANCE OF ENZYMES IN BIOLOGY

Enzymes play a significant role in variety of processes:

1. **Biological uses:** A large number of chemical reactions take place in a living cell. These reactions made to occur outside a living cell would require a very high temperature or would occur very slowly. These biological enzymes make the biochemical reactions occur at ordinary temperature and also at quick pace. For example, one molecule of enzyme urease can break down 30000 molecules of urea into carbon dioxide and ammonia in one second. In the absence of enzyme, this reaction would take years.

$$H_2N - C - NH_2 + H_2O \xrightarrow{\text{urease}} CO_2 + 2NH_3$$
urea   Water   Carbon dioxide Ammonia

2. **Physiology:** Enzymes present in stomach quickly and efficiently carry out the process of digestion. Enzymes are also important for respiration, nerve impulse transmission, blood clothing, etc; this enzymes are essential for carrying out biochemical processes.

3. **Medical diagnosis:** ELISA (enzyme linked immunosorbent assay) is used for detecting diseases like AIDS, Lyme disease.

4. **Medical treatment:** Enzyme streptokinase is used for dissolving blood clot formed inside blood vessels.

5. **Genetic engineering:** Enzyme like ligases and endonucleases are used in genetic engineering.

Enzymes work efficiently in association with various factors which enhance its activity, these factors may be:

Cofactors which are small non-protein inorganic molecule that carries out chemical reactions that cannot be performed by the standard 20 amino acids. **Examples** of **cofactors** include metal ions like iron and zinc.

Coenzymes which are organic molecules that are non-proteins and mostly derivatives of vitamins soluble in water by phosphorylation. Examples of coenzyme include thiamine pyrophosphate (TPP), flavin adenine dinucleotide (FAD), biotin

Apoenzyme is an inactive form of enzyme lacking the association of coenzyme and/or cofactors. Activation of the enzyme occurs upon binding of an organic or inorganic cofactor.

Holoenzyme is a complete and catalytically active form of enzyme. An apoenzyme together with its cofactor is holoenzyme. Examples of holoenzymes include DNA polymerase and RNA polymerase which contain multiple protein subunits (Fig. 5.9).

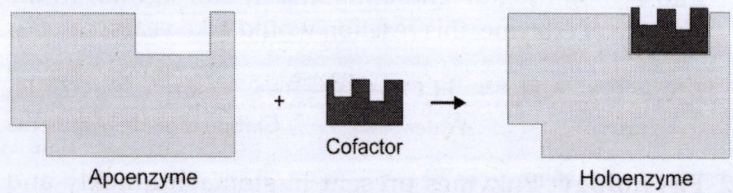

Fig. 5.9: Apoenzyme + Cofactor = Holoenzyme

RNA Catalysis

Riboenzymes are (RNA molecules that accelerate chemical reactions) the enzymes that happen to made up of RNA rather than protein. Two most important reactions of the cells catalysed by RNA are:

1. Splicing
2. Viral replication

Investigators studying origin of life have produced riboenzymes in the lab which are capable of catalyzing their own synthesis from monomers.

Application

1. Riboenzymes have been proposed and developed for the treatment of disease through gene therapy.
2. Synthetic riboenzyme has been developed and entered clinical testing for HIV infection.
3. Riboenzyme have been designed to target the hepatitis C virus.

KEY POINTS

- A catalyst influences the rate of a chemical reaction, usually without undergoing any change itself.
- Homogeneous catalysis reaction is one in which both the catalyst and the substances are in the same phase, i.e. either solid, liquid or gas.
- Heterogeneous catalysis reaction is one in which the catalyst is in a different phase from the substances on which it acts.
- An enzyme is a specialized protein produced with an organism which is capable of catalyzing a specific chemical reaction.
- All enzymes are proteins which are high molecular weight macromolecules.
- Active site: An enzyme has a distinct cavity or cleft in which the substrate is bound.
- Factors affecting enzyme action are temperature, pH, concentration of substrate and product concentration
- Mechanism of enzyme action: Two hypothesis 1. Lock and key hypothesis, 2. Induced fit hypothesis:
- Inhibition of enzyme action: Act in three different ways 1. Competitive inhibition, 2. Non-competitive inhibition 3. Allosteric inhibition

- Cofactors which are small non-protein inorganic molecule that carries out chemical reactions that cannot be performed by the standard 20 amino acids. Examples: Iron and zinc.
- Coenzymes which are organic molecules that are non-proteins and mostly derivatives of vitamins soluble in water by phosphorylation. Examples are thiamine pyrophosphate (TPP).
- Apoenzyme is an inactive form of enzyme lacking the association of coenzyme and/or cofactors. Activation of the enzyme occurs upon binding of an organic or inorganic cofactor.
- Holoenzyme is a complete and catalytically active form of enzyme. An apoenzyme together with its cofactor is holoenzyme. Examples: DNA polymerase and RNA polymerase.

PRACTICE QUESTIONS

Very Short Answer Type Questions

1. What is enzyme?
2. Give example of any enzyme which functions in body.
3. What is the function of oxireductases?
4. Give one example of transferases.
5. What is the function of hydrolases?
6. What is the function of lyases?

Short Answer Type Questions

1. What is active site?
2. Explain function of isomerase along with its example.
3. Explain the function of ligases along with its example.
4. How does temperature affect enzyme activity?
5. How does pH affect enzyme activity?
6. How does concentration of substrate influence enzymes?

Long Answer Type Questions

1. Explain the classification of enzymes.
2. How do enzymes catalyze reactions?
3. What are the factors affecting enzyme activity?
4. Explain mechanisms of enzymatic action.
5. Explain inhibition of enzymatic action.
6. What is enzyme kinetics? Explain using a graph (a) K_m (b) V_{max}.
7. Explain the importance of enzymes in biology.
8. Write a note on RNA catalysis.

Information Transfer Purpose

DNA: A DOUBLE STRANDED HELIX

After most biologists became convinced that DNA was the genetic material, a race was on to determine how the structure of this molecule could account for its role in heredity. By the beginning of the 1950, arrangement of covalent bonds in a nucleic acid polymer was well established and researchers focused on discovering the three-dimensional structure of DNA. Among the many scientists working on the problem were two scientists American James D. Watson and Englishman Francis Crick.

The brief but celebrated partnership soon solved the puzzle of DNA structure.

WATSON-CRICK MODEL OF DNA

1. The model says that DNA exists as a double helix. A DNA molecule has two unbranched polynucleotide strands. Each

polynucleotide strand or chain consists of a sequence of nucleotides linked together by phospodiester bonds. The polynucleotide strands are anti-parallel and seen in opposite direction.

2. The two strands are not coiled upon each other but the double strand is coiled upon itself around a common axis like spiral staircase with base pair forming steps while the backbone of the two strands form railing. Backbone is formed of sugar and phosphate.

3. base pairing is specific Adenine always pair with thymine and guanine pairs with cytosine, thus all base pair consists of one purine and one pyrimidine. Once the sequence of base in one strand of DNA double helix is known, the sequence of base in another strand can also be known because of specific base pairing. The two strands of DNA are said to be complementary. This is known as complementary base pairing.

4. The two polynucleotide strands are held together by hydrogen bonding between bases in opposite strands. Adenine and thymine are connected with two hydrogen bonds, guanine and cytosine are connected with three hydrogen bonds.

5. One end of strand is called 5′ end where fifth carbon of pentose sugar is free and the other end is called 3′ end where the third carbon of pentose is free.

6. At each base pair the strand turns 36°, one full turn of the helical strand (360°) would involve ten base pairs, i.e. one turn of 360 m° of helical strand has about ten nucleotides on each strand of DNA. The base pairs in DNA are stacked 3–4 Å apart. Thus pitch of DNA is 34 Å apart as ten base pairs occupy a distance of about 34 Å (Fig. 6.1).

Chargaff's Rule

In 1950, Chargaff found that in a DNA molecule:

1. Amount of purines and pyrimidines are equal.

$$A + G = T + C$$

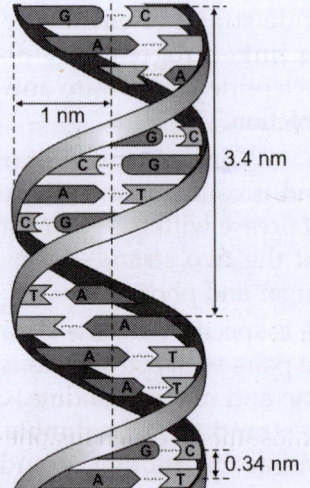

(a) Key features of DNA structure

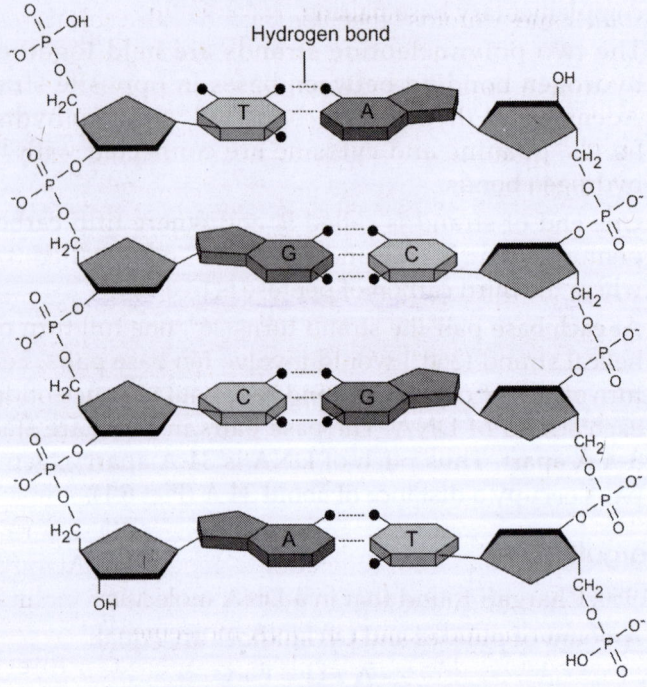

(b) Partial chemical structure

Fig. 6.1: Structure of DNA double Helix

2. Amount of adenine is equal to thymine and amount of guanine is always equal to cytosine

$$A = T \text{ and } G = C$$

3. Deoxyribose sugar and phosphate components occur in equal proportions.

Nucleosomes

Walter Flemming observed banded objects in the nuclei of stained eukaryote cells. He called the material chromosome which contains DNA plus the various proteins that package the DNA in a more compact form.

In humans, nucleus contains 46 chromosomes. The major protein of chromosomes is called histones. Histones are simple, basic proteins containing numerous lysine and Arginine amino acids whose positive charge allow the proteins to bind to negatively charged sugar phosphate backbone of DNA. Chromosomes unfolds when it is treated with a solution of low ionic strength. The extended chromosome looks like beads on string in a electron micrograph. The beads are DNA histone complex called nucleosome and the string is double stranded DNA. Each nucleosome consists of histone around which DNA is wrapped (Fig. 6.2).

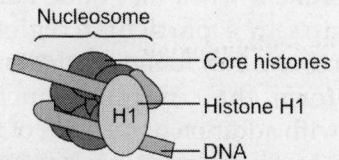

Fig. 6.2: Structure of nucleosome

GENETIC CODE

As DNA is a genetic material, it carries genetic information from cell to cell and from generation to generation. At this stage, an attempt will be made to determine in what manner the genetic information existed in DNA molecule.

As we know, DNA molecule is composed of three kind of components: (1) Phosphoric acid, (2) deoxyribose sugar, (3) nitrogenous base. Since the sugar phosphate forms the backbone of DNA and is always same, therefore, it is unlikely that this component of DNA carry the genetic information. Nitrogen bases, however, vary from one segment of DNA molecule to another, so the genetic information will depend on their sequence. These four DNA bases can be considered as four alphabets of DNA molecules.

George Gamow first proposed the basic structural unit of genetic code. The basic problem of genetic code is to indicate how information written in four letter language of nitrogenous base of DNA can be translated into twenty letter language of amino acids of proteins.

The group of nucleotides that specifies the amino acid is a code word or codon. The simplest possible code is a single code in which one nucleotide code for one amino acid, such a code is inadequate as only four amino acids can be specified. A doublet code, a code of two letters is also inadequate because it could specify only sixteen (4×4) amino acids (Fig. 6.3).

A triplet code, a code of three letters, could specify sixty four ($4 \times 4 \times 4$) amino acids. Therefore, it is likely that there are 64 triplet codes for 20 amino acids.

The first experimental evidence on support to the concept of triplet code was provided by Crick and coworkers in 1961. During the experiment when they added or deleted single or double base pairs in a particular region of DNA of T4 bacteriophage of *E. coli*, they found out that such bacteriophages ceased to perform their normal functions. However, bacteriophages with addition or deletion of three base pairs in DNA molecules had performed normal functions, from this experiment they concluded that a genetic code is in triplet form because the addition of one or four nucleotides has put the reading of the code out of order. While the addition of third nucleotides resulted in a return to the proper reading of the message.

Process for Making a Protein

Genes that provide instructions for proteins are expressed a two-step process.

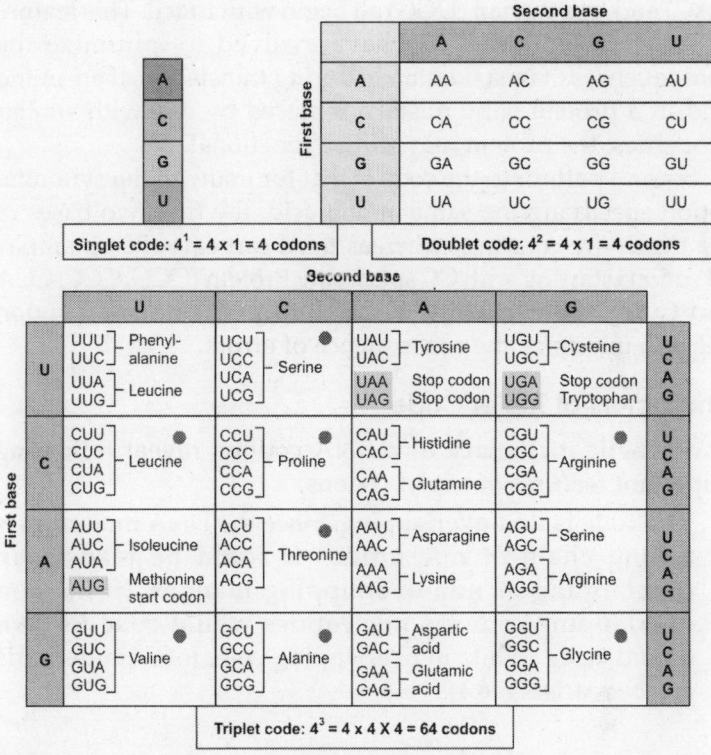

Fig. 6.3: Genetic code showing singlet, doublet and triplet code

1. In transcription the DNA sequences of a gene are rewritten in the RNA eukaryotes, the RNA must go through additional steps to become a messenger RNA (mRNA).

2. In translation the sequence of nuclcotides is the mRNA is translated into a sequence of amino acids in a polypeptides (protein chain).

Pattern to the Genetic Code

A notable pattern emerged when the genetic code was studied. First amino acids with similar structural properties tend to have related codons , thus aspartic acid codons (GAU and GAC) are similar to glutamic acid codons (GAA, GAG), similarly codons for aromatic acid phenylalaline (UAU, UUC), tyrosine (UUU,

UAC) and tryptophan (UGG) all begin with uracil. This feature of the code is thought to have evolved to minimize the consequences of mistakes made during translation. If an amino acid in a protein is by mistake replaced by one with similar properties, the protein may still be functional.

Second pattern to the code is that for many of the synonym codon specifying the same amino acid, the first two bases of the triplet are constant, whereas third can vary. For example, all codons starting with CC specifying Protein (CCU, CCC, CCA and CCG), this flexibility in the third nucleotide of a codon helps to minimize the consequence of errors.

Characters of Triplet Code

The genetic dictionary of mRNA codons reveal following important features of triplet codons.

1. **The code is non-overlapping:** Since the DNA molecules is a long chain of nucleotides it could be read in an overlapping or non-overlapping manner. In the non overlapping code six nucleotides would code for two amino acids. While in overlapping code four amino acids can be read (Fig. 6.4).

$$\frac{aa_1}{CAU} \quad \frac{aa_2}{GAU}$$

Non-overlapping code C, A, U and G are bases aa_1 and aa_2 are amino acids.

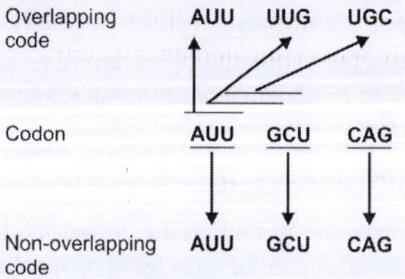

Fig. 6.4: Overlapping and non-overlapping code

Overlapping code: Studies on gene mutations show the code is non-overlapping type in the tobacco mosaic trees

(TMV) mutation of one base of mosaic acid results in alteration of only one single amino acid.

2. **The code is commaless:** The genetic code reads in an uninterrupted manner from one end of nucleic acid chain to another or are the bases (commas) between successive codons to code with commas can be represented as follows (x represent a base acting as comma):

UUU × CUC × GUA × UCC × ACC ——— Base

Phe   Leu   Val   Ser   Thr ——Amino acid

A commaless code would have no comma bases and can be represented as:

UUU   CUC   GUA   UCC ——— Base

Phe   Leu   Val   Thr ——— Amino acid

All the available evidence indicates that the code is commaless. The work of of Khorana and his associate gave clear evidence of commaless code.

3. **Code has polarity:** If a gene is to specify the same protein repeatedly it is essential the code must have fixed start and end points. These points are the indication and termination codons respectively. The code must be read in a fixed direction. In other words, code must have polarity. The available evidence indicates code is read in $5' \rightarrow 3'$ direction in mRNA. The polypeptides chain is synthesized in $N \rightarrow C$ direction, from amino (NH_2) terminal to carboxyl (COOH) terminal.

4. **Codons and anticodons:** During translation the codons of mRNA pair with complementary anticodons of tRNA. Since mRNA is read in polar manner in the $5' \rightarrow 3'$ directions, the codons are written on $5' \rightarrow 3'$ direction. The codon AUG is written as 5' AUG 3'. Often to make things simpler, anticodons are written $3' \rightarrow 5'$ directions so as to bring easier correlation between codon and anticodon bases.

Codon (mRNA) – 5' AUG 3'

Anticodon (tRNA) – 3' UAC 5'

5. **Initiation codon:** The starting amino acid in syntheses of most proteins chain is methionine (eukryotes) or N. formyl

methionine (Prokryotes). It is find to initiation sites containing AUG codon. This codon is, therefore, called the initiation codon. Less often GUG also function as initiation codon in bacterial protein.

6. **Termination codon:** Three of 64 codons do not specify any tRNA and are hence called nonsense codons. These codons are (UAG) amber, UAA (ochre) and UGA (opal or umber), since they bring about termination of polypeptide chain synthesis, they are also called termination codons.

7. **The code is degenerate:** There are 64 possible codons in a triplet code of which 61 take part to code amino acids. Since only 20 amino acids take part in protein synthesis, it is obvious that there are many more codons types, as a result there are multiple codons for most amino acids. For example: There are six codons for serine, four for glycine and two for lysine. Because of the existence of several codons for most amino acids, the genetic code is said to be degenerate.

Different codons that specify the same amino acid are known as synonymous codons. The degeneracy of genetic code minimises the effect of mutations since changing a single nucleotide often results in a codon that still specifies the same amino acid. In a standard genetic code, the only amino acids with single codon are methionine and tryptophan.

Wobble hypothesis: The triplet code is a degenerate one with many more codons that the number of amino acid types coded. An explanation for this degeneracy is provided by the Wobble hypothesis proposed by Crick (1966). Since there are 61 codons specifying amino acids the cell should contain 61 different tRNA molecules each with a different anticodons but the number of tRNA molecules types discovered is much less than 61. This implies that the anticodon of some tRNA read more than one codon in mRNA.

According to the Wobble hypothesis, only the first two positions of the triplet codon on mRNA have a precise pairing with the basis of the tRNA anticodon. The pairing of the third position bases of the codon may be ambiguous and varies according to the nucleotide present in this position. Thus a single tRNA type is able to recognize two or more codons differing only in the third base. For example, anticodon UCG of serine tRNA recognizes two codons AGC and AGU. The bonding between UCG and AGU follows the usual Watson-Crick pairing. In UCG and AGU pairing hydrogen bonding takes place between G and U which is different from the usual Watson-Crick pairing where G pairs with C and A with U. Such interaction between the third base is referred to as 'Wobble pairing'.

mRNA codon (Serine)	5' AGC 3'	5' AGU 3'
tRNA anticodon	3' UCG 5'	3' UCG 5'

8. **The code is universal:** The genetic code is valid for all organisms ranging from bacteria to man. It is essentially same for all organisms and so it is said to be universal. The universality of the code was demonstrated by Marshall and Nirenberg who found *E. coli* (bacteria), *Xenops laevis* (amphibian) and guinea pig (mammal) use almost the same code, this showed that the code is essentially universal.

Techniques of Genetic Engineering

New techniques have been developed to manipulate the genetic material. Genetic engineering started in 1993 by combining a gene from a bacterium with the plasmid of *E.coli*. Genetic engineering techniques have been used for many purposes useful for mankind. This new techniques of genetic engineering are known as recombinant DNA technology which deals with manipulation of genetic material by man *in vitro*.

Recombinant DNA Technology

It involves two basic processes:

1. Formation of recombinant DNA.
2. Introduction of recombinant DNA into an appropriate host.

Recombinant DNA is formed by combining DNA from different organisms. For example, insulin gene cut off from rat's DNA and linked to bacterial plasmid gives recombinant DNA.

Denaturation and renaturation are the two properties which help in the formation of recombinant DNA. Denaturation is the separation of strands of DNA by breaking of hydrogen bonds in heating. Renaturation is the reunion of complementary strands to form double helix on cooling.

Tools of Recombinant DNA Technology

Three types of biological tools are used in synthesis of recombinant DNA. These include:

1. Enzymes
2. Vectors DNA
3. Passenger DNA

Enzymes

Many kind of enzymes are used in genetic engineering. These include:

1. Lysing enzyme: These are used to open up the cells to get DNA for genetic experiments. Lysozyme is commonly used to dissolve the bacterial cell wall.

2. Clearing enzymes: These are used to break DNA molecule. These are of three kinds:

   a. Exonucleases: Which cut off nucleotide in 5′ or 3′ end of DNA molecule.

   b. Endonucleases: Which cut off DNA molecule at any part except ends.

   c. Restriction endonucleases: Which cut off DNA duplex at specific point in such a way that single stranded free ends project from each fragment of DNA duplex. The single stranded free ends are called 'sticky ends' because they can join similar complementary ends of DNA fragment from other source and can be said as a molecular scissors EcoR1 is commonly used restriction enzyme.

3. Synthesizing enzymes: These enzymes play a role in the synthesis of DNA strands on suitable templates. These are of two types:

   a. Reverse transcriptase: Which helps in the synthesis of complementary DNA strand on RNA template.

b. DNA polymerase: Which helps in the syntheses of complementary DNA strand on DNA template.

4. Joining enzymes: They help in scaling gaps in DNA fragment which are otherwise formed by complementary base pairing. They are the molecular glues. They join DNA fragments by forming phosphodiester bonds.

5. Alkaline phosphatases: These cut off phosphate group from 5' end of linearised circular DNA to check its recircularization.

Vehicle of Vector DNA

DNA used as a carrier for transferring fragment of foreign DNA into a suitable host is called vehicle DNA. It is also called a gene carrier. The desired gene is introduced in a vector where recombinant DNA (rDNA) is formed. The vector carrying rDNA divides, thereby forming the several copies of rDNA. Five types of DNA are used as vehicles:

1. Plasmid DNA
2. Bacteriophage DNA
3. DNA of plant and animal virus
4. Transposons (jumping genes)
5. Artificial DNA

Plasmids and bacteriophage DNA are commonly used vehicles.

1. **Plasmids:** These are small double stranded, closed circular symbiotic DNA molecules that naturally occurs in bacteria, outside bacterial chromosome and are regarded as extra chromosomal DNA. A bacteria cell may have one or many copies of plasmids. They are inherited from parent bacterial cell to daughter cells and have the capability for self-replication the cytoplasm of bacteria.

   Another feature of plasmids is the presence of specific restriction site where the enzyme restriction endonucleases make a cut so that foreign DNA segment may be joined to the plasmid. These are resistant to antibodies.

2. **Bacteriophage vectors:** They are the virus that infect bacteria by introducing their DNA into bacterial cell. The

injected DNA of virus integrates into bacterial chromosome. This viral DNA multiplies with bacterial chromosome as prophage.

Passenger DNA: It is the DNA which is transferred from one organism into another by combining it with the vehicle DNA. Three types of DNA are used as passenger DNA.

a. *Complementary or copy DNA (cDNA):* It is synthesized on RNA template with the help of reverse transcriptase enzyme and necessary nucleotides. The DNA strand is isolated from the hybrid RNA-DNA complex by using alkaline phosphates enzymes. A complementary DNA strand is then synthesized on the isolated single stranded DNA template with the help of DNA polymerase. The cDNA duplex so formed can be joined to vehicle DNA for introduction into cell.

b. *Synthetic DNA (sDNA):* It is synthesized with the help of DNA polymers on DNA templates.

Process of Recombinant DNA Technology

It involves the integration of passenger DNA to vehicle DNA. The passenger DNA is taken out of the cell by lysing with a suitable enzyme. The DNA is isolated from other cell contents, then both passenger and vehicle DNA are cleaned by using the same restriction endonuclease so that they have complementary sticky ends. They are mixed under suitable conditions. Their complementary sticky ends pair and ends are sealed with ligase. This produces a recombinant DNA.

Earlier *E. coli* was used as a test for recombinant DNA but now *Bacillus subtilis* and yeast are also used. Three methods are used for introducing recombinant DNA into the host. These are:

1. **Transformation:** It is a process in which cell takes up naked DNA fragment from the environment incorporates it into the own chromosomal DNA and expresses the tract controlled by incoming DNA. For example, plasmid of bacterium *E. coli* and insulin gene of rat are isolated and sliced with restriction endonuclease to produce complimentary sticky ends in both DNA segments. At free

sticky ends the plasmid DNA and rat DNA undergo complementary pairing, gaps are sealed with ligase forming a circular DNA from two different DNA segments. This recombinant DNA is then introduced into a bacterium to produce several copies of recombinant DNA and finally insulin is extracted.

2. **Transduction:** Transfer of DNA from one organism to another through a bacteriophage is called transduction. For example, genes were transferred from bacterium *E. coli* into human cells through intermediate virus. Cells of culture were taken from a person who lacked the enzyme (beta-galactosidase) to digest lactose. Since *E. coli* had this gene for synthesis of enzyme so these were made to enter human cells in culture through DNA bacteriophage and started functioning in them and ability to produce the enzyme started.

3. **Vector less gene transfer:** Several alternatives approaches have been made to introduce the recombinant DNA into recipient cells without involving carrier molecules.

In biology a clone is a group of individual's cells or organisms descended from one progenitor. This means the members of clone are generally identical. The use of word clone has been extended to recombinant DNA technology, which has provided scientists with the ability to produce many copies of a single fragment of DNA, such as a gene, creating identical copies that construct a DNA clone by the method explained above.

KEY POINTS

- Watson-Crick Model of DNA: The model says that DNA exists as a double helix.
- A DNA molecule has two unbranched polynucleotide strands. Each polynucleotide strand or chain consists of a sequence of nucleotides linked together by phosphodiester bonds.
- Base pairing is specific adenine always pair with thymine and guanine pairs with cytosine.

- The two strands of DNA are complementary.
- The two polynucleotide strands are held together by hydrogen bonding.
- In humans, nucleus contains 46 chromosomes.
- The major protein of chromosomes is called histones.
- Histones are simple, basic proteins containing numerous lysine and arginine amino acids whose positive charge allows the proteins to bind to negatively charged sugar phosphate backbone of DNA.
- DNA molecule is composed of three kind of components: (1) Phosphoric acid, (2) deoxyribose sugar, (3) nitrogenous base.
- Characters of triplet code:
  1. The code is nonoverlapping
  2. The code is commaless
  3. Code has polarity
  4. The code is degenerative
- Initiation codon: The starting amino acid in syntheses of most proteins chain is methionine (eukryotes) or N. formyl methionine (prokryotes).
- AUG is called the initiation codon.
- Termination codon: Also called nonsense codons. These codons are (UAG) amber, UAA (ochre) and UGA (opal or umber) since they bring about termination of polypeptide chain synthesis, they are also called termination codons.
- The code is universal: The genetic code is valid for all organisms ranging from bacteria to man.
- Tools of recombinant DNA technology are
  1. Enzymes
  2. Vectors DNA
  3. Passenger DNA
- Vehicle of vector DNA: DNA used as a carrier for transferring fragment of foreign DNA into a suitable host is called vehicle DNA. It is also called a gene carrier.

- Five types of DNA are used as vehicles:
  1. Plasmid DNA
  2. Bacteriophage DNA
  3. DNA of plant and animal virus
  4. Transposons (jumping genes)
  5. Artificial DNA.
- Transformation: It is a process in which cell takes up naked DNA fragment from the environment incorporates it into the own chromosomal DNA and expresses the tract controlled by incoming DNA.
- Transduction: Transfer of DNA from one organism to another through a bacteriophage is called transduction.

PRACTICE QUESTIONS

Very Short Answer Type Questions

1. Give example of (a) initiation codon, (b) termination codon.
2. What is genetic code?
3. Why is doublet code inadequate?
4. What is transcription?
5. What is translation?
6. Who gave the double helix model of DNA?
7. What is complementary base pairing?
8. How many hydrogen bonds are used to connect adenine and thymine?

Short Answer Type Questions

1. What is triplet genetic code?
2. What do you mean by code is non-overlapping?
3. Explain code polarity.
4. Differences between codon and anti-codon.
5. Explain the code is degenerate.
6. What are nucleosomes?
7. What is Chargaff's rule?
8. What are plasmids?

Long Answer Type Questions

1. Give the characteristics of genetic codon.
2. What do you mean by the code is universal?
3. Explain Wobble hypothesis?
4. Explain the structure of nucleosomes along with its diagram.
5. Why is DNA molecule compared to spiraling staircase? Explain using the Watson-Crick model of DNA.

Macromolecular Analysis

A **macromolecule** is a very large molecule, such as protein, commonly created by the polymerization of smaller subunits (monomers). The term *macromolecule (macro- + molecule)* was coined by Nobel laureate Hermann Staudinger in 1920.

"Macromolecule is a molecule of high relative molecular mass, the structure of which essentially comprises the multiple repetition of units derived, actually or conceptually, from molecules of low relative molecular mass."

They are typically composed of thousands of atoms or more. The most common macromolecules are biopolymers like

1. Nucleic acids

2. Proteins

3. Carbohydrates

4. Lipids

Synthetic macromolecules include common plastics and synthetic fibers

LINEAR BIOPOLYMERS

All living organisms are dependent on three essential biopolymers for their biological functions: DNA, RNA and proteins. Each of these molecules is required for life since each plays a distinct, indispensable role in the cell. The simple summary is that DNA makes RNA, and then RNA makes proteins.

DNA FOR ENCODING INFORMATION

DNA is an information storage macromolecule that encodes the complete set of instructions (the genome) that are required to assemble, maintain, and reproduce every living organism.

DNA and RNA are both capable of encoding genetic information, because there are biochemical mechanisms which read the information coded within a DNA or RNA sequence and use it to generate a specified protein.

PROTEINS FOR CATALYSIS

Proteins are functional macromolecules responsible for catalysing the biochemical reactions that sustain life. Proteins carry out all functions of an organism, for example, photosynthesis, neural function, vision, and movement.

RNA IS MULTIFUNCTIONAL

RNA is multifunctional, its primary function is to encode proteins, according to the instructions within a cell's DNA. They control and regulate many aspects of protein synthesis in eukaryotes.

RNA encodes genetic information that can be translated into the amino acid sequence of proteins, as evidenced by the messenger RNA molecules present within every cell, and the RNA genomes of a large number of viruses. The single-stranded nature of RNA, together with tendency for rapid breakdown and a lack of repair systems, means that RNA is not so well suited for the long-term storage of genetic information as is DNA.

HIERARCHY OF PROTEIN STRUCTURE

Linderstrom-Lang (1952) first proposed that there is hierarchy of protein structure with four, namely primary, secondary, tertiary, and quaternary.

1. **Primary structure** is the basic level of the hierarchy and is the particular linear sequence of amino acids that comprises one polypeptide chain.
2. **Secondary structure** is the next 'level up' from the primary structure and is the regular folding of regions within one polypeptide chain into particular structural patterns. Secondary structures are usually held together by hydrogen bonds between the carbonyl oxygen and the amide hydrogen of the peptide bond.
3. **Tertiary structure** is the next 'level up' from the secondary structure and is the particular three-dimensional arrangement of all the amino acids in one polypeptide chain. This structure is usually the native, and active, conformation and is held together by multiple noncovalent interactions.
4. **Quaternary structure** is the next 'level up' from the tertiary structure and is the particular spatial arrangement, and interactions, between two or more polypeptide chains.

The implications of this hierarchy are that:

1. Each level of the hierarchy is 'held together' by characteristic interactions and forces.
2. Higher levels of structure in the hierarchy are composed of the structural entities of the lower levels shown in Fig. 7.1.

FUNCTIONS OF PROTEINS

Protein is an important substance found in every cell in the human body. In fact, except for water, protein is the most abundant substance in your body. This protein is manufactured by your body utilizing the dietary protein you consume. It is used in many vital processes and thus needs to be consistently

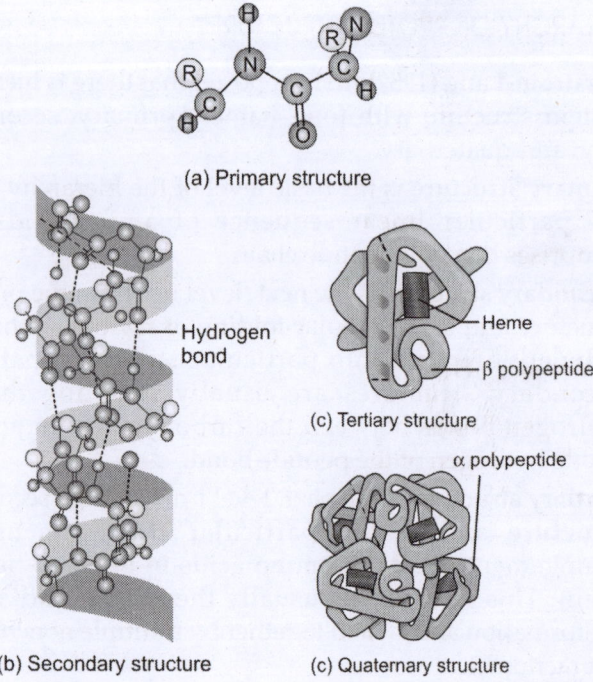

(a) Primary structure

Hydrogen bond

Heme

β polypeptide

(c) Tertiary structure

α polypeptide

(b) Secondary structure

(c) Quaternary structure

Fig. 7.1: Protein hierarchy showing primary, secondary, tertiary and quaternary structure

replaced. You can accomplish this by regularly consuming foods that contain protein.

ENZYMES

Enzymes are proteins that increase the rate of chemical reactions in the body. In fact, most of the necessary chemical reactions in the body would not efficiently proceed without enzymes. For example, one type of enzyme functions as an aid in digesting large protein, carbohydrate and fat molecules into smaller molecules, while another assists the creation of DNA.

Enzymes are proteins that speed up chemical reactions in the body and **hormones**, like insulin, are proteins that regulate the activity of cells or organs.

TRANSPORTATION AND STORAGE OF MOLECULES

Protein is a major element in transportation of certain molecules. For example, hemoglobin is a protein that transports oxygen throughout the body. Protein is also sometimes used to store certain molecules. Ferritin is an example of a protein that combines with iron for storage in the liver. Some proteins **transport** materials throughout your body, such as hemoglobin, which is the oxygen-transporting protein found in your **red blood cells.**

Receptor Proteins

These proteins are used in intercellular **communication**. In this animation you can see the hormone binding to the receptor. This causes the receptor proteins release a signal to perform some action.

Proteins as Structural Elements

They do most of the work in cells and are required for the **structure, function**, and regulation of the **body's** tissues and organs. **Proteins** are made up of hundreds or thousands of smaller units called amino acids, which are attached to one another in long chains. These **proteins** provide **structure** and support for cells.

Proteins can be described according to their large range of functions in the body, listed in Table 7.1.

KEY POINTS

- A macromolecule is a very large molecule, such as protein, commonly created by the polymerization of smaller subunits (monomers).
- The term macromolecule (macro + molecule) was coined by Nobel laureate Hermann Staudinger in 1920.
- "Macromolecule is a molecule of high relative molecular mass, the structure of which essentially comprises the multiple repetition of units derived, actually or conceptually, from molecules of low relative molecular mass".

Table 7.1 Functions of proteins, their description and example

S.No	Function	Description	Example
1.	Antibody	Antibodies bind to specific foreign particles, such as viruses and bacteria, to help protect the body.	Immunoglobulin G (IgG)
2.	Enzyme	Enzymes carry out almost all of the thousands of chemical reactions that take place in cells. They also assist with the formation of new molecules by reading the genetic information stored in DNA.	Phenylalanine-hydroxylase
3.	Messenger	Messenger proteins, such as some types of hormones, transmit signals to coordinate biological processes between different cells, tissues, and organs.	Growth hormone
4.	Structural component	These proteins provide structure and support for cells. On a larger scale, they also allow the body to move.	Actin
5.	Transport/ storage	These proteins bind and carry atoms and small molecules within cells and throughout the body.	Ferritin

- The most common macromolecules are biopolymers like
  1. Nucleic acids
  2. Proteins
  3. Carbohydrates
  4. Lipids
- DNA is an information storage macromolecule.
- Proteins are functional macromolecules responsible for catalysing the biochemical reactions.
- RNA is multifunctional, its primary function is to encode proteins.

- Linderstrom-Lang (1952) first proposed that there is hierarchy of protein structure with four, namely primary, secondary, tertiary, and quaternary.
- Primary structure is the basic level of the hierarchy and is the particular linear sequence of amino acids that comprises one polypeptide chain.
- Secondary structure is the next 'level up' from the primary structure and is the regular folding of regions within one polypeptide chain into particular structural patterns. Secondary structures are usually held together by hydrogen bonds.
- Tertiary structure is the next 'level up' from the secondary structure and is the particular three-dimensional arrangement of all the amino acids in one polypeptide chain held together by multiple noncovalent interactions.
- Quaternary structure is the next 'level up' from the tertiary structure.
- Enzymes are proteins that speed up chemical reactions in the body and hormones, like insulin, are proteins that regulate the activity of cells or organs.

PRACTICE QUESTIONS

Very Short Answer Type Questions

1. What is a macromolecule?
2. What is the basic unit of proteins?
3. Give one example of hormonal protein.
4. Give the name of protein that fights against diseases.
5. Give example of enzymatic proteins which help in digestion.

Short Answer Type Questions

1. What is meant by primary structure of proteins?
2. Explain (a) α-helix (b) β-pleated sheets in secondary protein structure.
3. What is meant by tertiary structure of proteins?

4. How do proteins act as enzymes?
5. How do proteins help in transportation of substances in the body?

Long Answer Type Questions

1. Explain in detail primary, secondary, tertiary and quaternary structure of proteins.
2. Write in detail the function of proteins.

Metabolism

ENERGY TRANSFORMATION IN BIOLOGICAL SYSTEMS

The sun is the primary source of energy for living organisms. Some living organisms like plants need sunlight directly while other organisms like humans can acquire energy from the sun indirectly. There is, however, evidence that some bacteria can thrive in harsh environments like Antarctica as evidence by the blue-green algae beneath thick layers of ice in the lakes. No matter what the type of living species, all living organisms must capture, transduce, store, and use energy to live. Plants trap this energy from the sunlight and undergo photosynthesis, effectively converting solar energy into chemical energy. To transfer the energy once again, animals will feed on plants and use the energy of digested plant materials to create biological macromolecules.

135

LAWS OF THERMODYNAMICS AS RELATED TO BIOLOGY

Definition

The laws of thermodynamics are important unifying principles of biology. These principles govern the chemical processes (metabolism) in all biological organisms.

The First Law of Thermodynamics, also known as the law of conservation of energy, states that energy can neither be created nor destroyed. It may change from one form to another, but the energy in a closed system remains constant.

The Second Law of Thermodynamics states that when energy is transferred, there will be less energy available at the end of the transfer process than at the beginning. Due to **entropy**, which is the measure of disorder in a closed system, all of the available energy will not be useful to the organism. Entropy increases as energy is transferred.

In addition to the laws of thermodynamics, the cell theory, gene theory, evolution, and homeostasis form the basic principles that are the foundation for the study of life.

FIRST LAW OF THERMODYNAMICS IN BIOLOGICAL SYSTEMS

All biological organisms require energy to survive. In a closed system, such as the universe, this energy is not consumed but transformed from one form to another. Cells, for example, perform a number of important processes. These processes require energy. In photosynthesis, the energy is supplied by the sun. Light energy is absorbed by cells in plant leaves and converted to chemical energy. The chemical energy is stored in the form of glucose, which is used to form complex carbohydrates necessary to build plant mass. The energy stored in glucose can also be released through cellular respiration. This process allows plant and animal organisms to access the energy stored in carbohydrates, lipids, and other macromolecules through the production of ATP. This energy is needed to perform cell functions such as DNA replication, mitosis, meiosis, cell movement, endocytosis, exocytosis, and apoptosis.

SECOND LAW OF THERMODYNAMICS IN BIOLOGICAL SYSTEMS

As with other biological processes, the transfer of energy is not 100% efficient. In photosynthesis, for example, not all of the light energy is absorbed by the plant. Some energy is reflected and some is lost as heat. The loss of energy to the surrounding environment results in an increase of disorder or entropy. Unlike plants and other photosynthetic organisms, animals cannot generate energy directly from the sunlight. They must consume plants or other animal organisms for energy. The higher up an organism is on the food chain, the less available energy it receives from its food sources. Much of this energy is lost during metabolic processes performed by the producers and primary consumers that are eaten. Therefore, much less energy is available for organisms in higher trophic levels. The lower the available energy, the less number of organisms can be supported. This is why there are more producers than consumers in an ecosystem.

Living systems require constant energy input to maintain their highly ordered state. Cells, for example, are highly ordered and have low entropy. In the process of maintaining this order, some energy is lost to the surroundings or transformed. So while cells are ordered, the processes performed to maintain that order result in an increase in entropy in the cell's/organism's surroundings. The transfer of energy causes entropy in the universe to increase.

Exothermic and Endothermic Versus Endergonic and Exergonic Reactions

Many chemical reactions release energy in the form of heat, light, or sound. These are exothermic reactions. Exothermic reactions may occur spontaneously and result in higher randomness or entropy ($\Delta S > 0$) of the system. They are denoted by a negative heat flow (heat is lost to the surroundings) and decrease in enthalpy ($\Delta H < 0$). In the lab, exothermic reactions produce heat or may even be explosive.

There are other chemical reactions that must absorb energy in order to proceed. These are endothermic reactions.

Endothermic reactions cannot occur spontaneously. Work must be done in order to get these reactions to occur. When endothermic reactions absorb energy, a temperature drop is measured during the reaction. Endothermic reactions are characterized by positive heat flow (into the reaction) and an increase in enthalpy ($+\Delta H$).

Examples of Endothermic and Exothermic Processes

Photosynthesis is an example of an endothermic chemical reaction. In this process, plants use the energy from the sun to convert carbon dioxide and water into glucose and oxygen. This reaction requires 15MJ of energy (sunlight) for every kilogram of glucose that is produced

$$\text{Sunlight} + 6CO_2(g) + H_2O(l) \longrightarrow C_6H_{12}O_6 + 6O_2(g)$$

Respiration is an example of exothermic reaction.

$$C_6H_{12}O_6 + 6O_2 \longrightarrow 6CO_2 + 6H_2O + \text{Energy}$$

ENDOTHERMIC VS EXOTHERMIC COMPARISON

Here's a quick summary of the differences between endothermic and exothermic reactions (Table 8.1).

Table 8.1 Differences between endothermic and exothermic reactions

S.No	Endothermic	Exothermic
1.	Heat is absorbed (feels cold)	Heat is released (feels warm)
2.	Energy must be added for reaction to occur	Reaction occurs spontaneously
3.	Disorder decreases ($\Delta S < 0$)	Entropy increases ($\Delta S > 0$)
4.	Increase in enthalpy ($+\Delta H$)	Decrease in enthalpy ($-\Delta H$)

ENDERGONIC AND EXERGONIC REACTIONS

Endothermic and exothermic reactions refer to the absorption or release of heat. There are other types of energy which may be produced or absorbed by a chemical reaction. Examples include light and sound. In general, reactions involving energy may be classified as endergonic or exergonic, An endothermic reaction is an example of an **endergonic reaction**. An exothermic reaction is an example of an **exergonic reaction**.

Important Points

1. Endothermic and exothermic reactions are chemical reactions that absorb and release heat, respectively.

2. A good example of an endothermic reaction is photosynthesis. Combustion is an example of an exothermic reaction.

3. The categorization of a reaction as endo- or exothermic depends on the net heat transfer. In any given reaction, heat is both absorbed and released. For example, energy must be input into a combustion reaction to start it (lighting a fire with a match), but then more heat is released than was required.

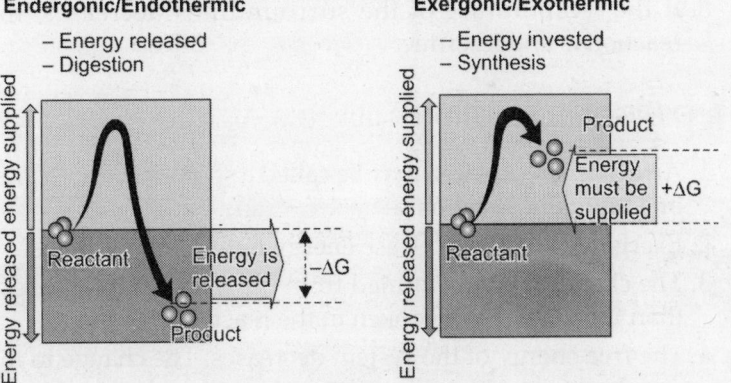

Endergonic vs. exergonic reactions

Endergonic/Endothermic
– Energy released
– Digestion

Exergonic/Exothermic
– Energy invested
– Synthesis

AP biology ΔG = changes in free energy = ability to do work

Fig. 8.1: Difference between exergonic and endergonic reactions

Endergonic and exergonic are two types of chemical reactions or processes in thermochemistry or physical chemistry. The names describe what happens to energy during the reaction. The classifications are related to endothermic and exothermic reactions, except endergonic and exergonic describe what happens with any form of energy, while endothermic and exothermic relate only to heat or thermal energy.

ENDERGONIC REACTIONS

1. An endergonic reactions may also be called an unfavorable reaction or nonspontaneous reaction. The reaction requires more energy than you get from it.
2. Endergonic reactions absorb energy from the surroundings.
3. The chemical bonds that are formed from the reaction are weaker than the chemical bonds that were broken.
4. The free energy of the system increases. The change in the standard Gibbs Free Energy (G) of an endergonic reaction is positive (greater than 0).
5. The change in entropy (S) decreases.
6. Endergonic reactions are not spontaneous.
7. Examples of endergonic reactions include endothermic reactions, such as photosynthesis and the melting of ice into liquid water.
8. If the temperature of the surroundings decreases, the reaction is endothermic.

EXERGONIC REACTIONS

1. An exergonic reaction may be called a spontaneous reaction or a favorable reaction.
2. Exergonic reactions release energy to the surroundings.
3. The chemical bonds formed from the reaction are stronger than those that were broken in the reactants.
4. The free energy of the system decreases. The change in the standard Gibbs Free Energy (G) of an exergonic reaction is negative (less than 0).
5. The change in entropy (S) increases. Another way to look at it is that the disorder or randomness of the system increases.
6. Exergonic reactions occur spontaneously (no outside energy is required to start them).
7. Examples of exergonic reactions include exothermic reactions, such as mixing sodium and chlorine to make table salt, combustion, and chemiluminescence (light is the energy that is released).

8. If the temperature of the surroundings increases, the reaction is exothermic.

Concept of K_{eq} and its Relation to Standard Free Energy. Equilibrium Constant and ΔG

At equilibrium the ΔG for a reversible reaction is equal to zero. K_{eq} relates the concentrations of all substances in the reaction at equilibrium. Therefore, we can write (through a more advanced treatment of thermodynamics) the following equation:

$$\Delta G\circ = -RT \ln K_{eq}$$

The variable R is the ideal gas constant (8.314 J/K • mol), T is the Kelvin temperature, and ln K_{eq} is the natural logarithm of the equilibrium constant.

When K_{eq} is large, the products of the reaction are favored and the negative sign in the equation means that the ΔG∘ is negative which indicates the reaction is a spontaneous reaction. When K_{eq} is small, the reactants of the reaction are favored. The natural logarithm of a number less than one is negative and so the sign of ΔG∘ is positive which indicates reaction is non-spontaneous and at equilibrium G = 0. The relationship of ΔG∘ to K_{eq} is summarized below.

Relationship of ΔG∘ and K_{eq}

$K_{eq} > 1$ positive Products are favored at equilibrium.

$K_{eq} = 1$ Reactants and products are equally favored.

$K_{eq} < 1$ negative Reactants are favored at equilibrium.

What Is a Spontaneous Reaction?

Imagine you are walking past a natural waterfall. The water that tumbles downhill does so of its own accord and does not need any help from levees or dams. Now imagine something even more common place—taking a nice, cold soda out of your fridge and putting it down next to your computer. After a while, the soda becomes room temperature; again, without any intervention on your part.

From this, we can define a **spontaneous reaction** as a reaction that occurs in a given set of conditions without intervention. A spontaneous reaction proceeds to completion without any outside help.

Just because a reaction is spontaneous, it does not automatically imply that these reactions occur instantaneously. An example of this is when iron nails rust due to constant exposure to moisture — this process does not occur overnight, but can take days or months. Still, the process does not need any outside intervention to occur.

SPONTANEOUS REACTIONS AND ENTROPY

Let us think about it this way: Where do you spend more effort, cleaning your house or making a mess? In general, we spend more effort and energy cleaning our houses, and if we miss a week or two of cleaning, then it easily becomes messy. We can say that making a mess is definitely a more spontaneous process.

According to the **Second Law of Thermodynamics**, a reaction is spontaneous if the overall entropy, or disorder, increases. If we go back to our cleaning the house analogy, when our home becomes messy, then the entropy increases. The mess that accumulates is a spontaneous reaction, and as a result, the entropy increases.

If the overall entropy change, represented as **dS**, increases, then the reaction is spontaneous.

In a spontaneous reaction, just because the overall change in entropy is positive does not mean that the entropy of the systems and surroundings should always *both* be positive. As long as the positive entropy of either the system or surroundings compensates for the negative entropy change of the other, then the reaction will be spontaneous.

ATP AS ENERGY CURRENCY

The nucleotide coenzyme **adenosine triphosphate** (ATP) is the most important **form of chemical energy** in all cells (Fig. 8.2).

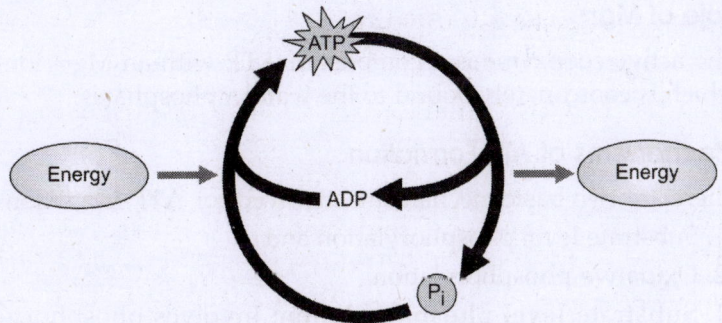

Fig. 8.2: Structure of ATP

ATP is a nucleoside triphosphate containing adenine, ribose, and three phosphate groups (Fig. 8.3).

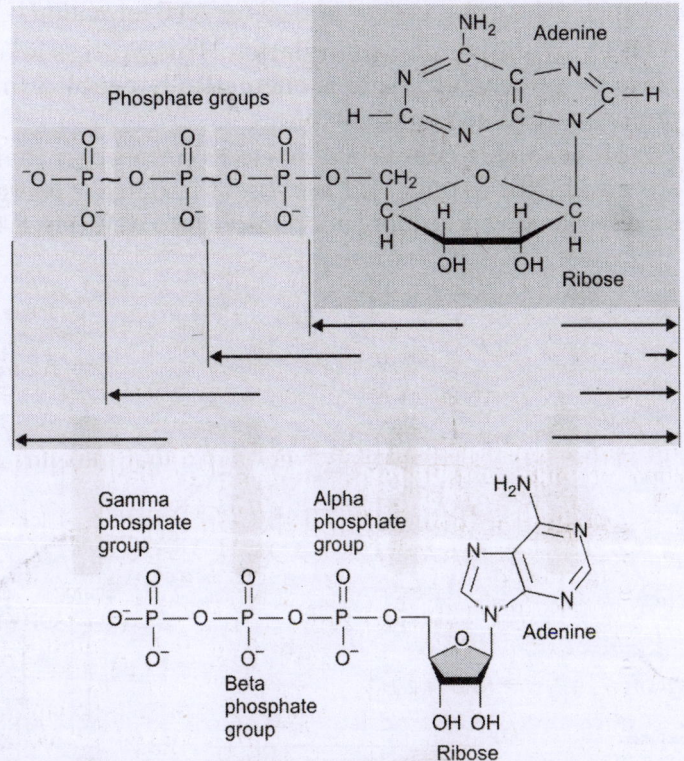

Fig. 8.3: Structure of ATP along with nucleoside triphosphate containing adenine, ribose, and three phosphate groups

Role of Mg++

The active coenzyme is a complex of ATP with an Mg^{2+} ion, which is coordinately bound to the β and γ phosphates.

Mechanisms of ATP Formation

There are two basic mechanisms involved for ATP formation:

1. Substrate level phosphorylation and
2. Oxidative phosphorylation

1. **Substrate level phosphorylation:** Involves phosphorylation of ADP to form ATP at the expense of the energy of the parent substrate molecule without involving the electron transport chain.

   Substrate is a high energy compound as compared to the product, the surplus energy is used for ATP formation.

2. **ATP by oxidative phosphorylation:** This process takes place in mitochondria and is energetically coupled to a proton gradient over a membrane.

   The H^+ gradients established by electron transport chain are used by the enzyme *ATP synthase* as a source of energy for direct linking of an inorganic phosphate to ADP (Fig. 8.4).

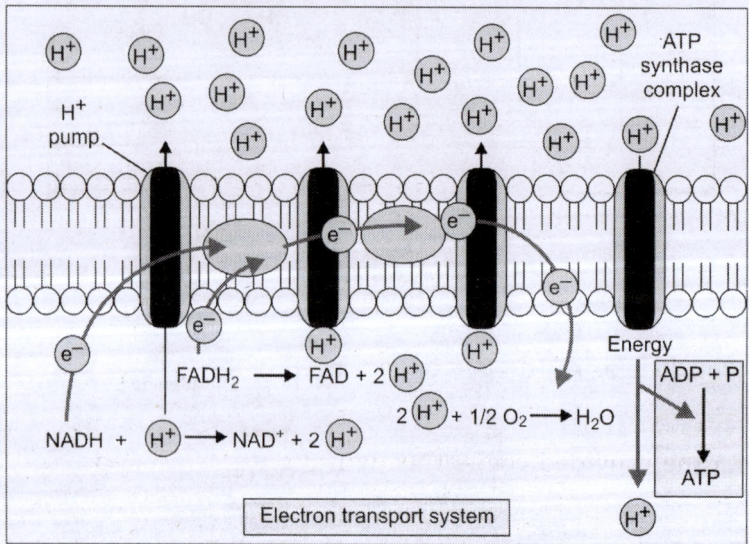

Fig. 8.4: Electron transport System

Energy of Hydrolysis

1. Energy is usually liberated from the ATP molecule to do work in the cell by a reaction that removes one of the phosphate-oxygen groups, leaving adenosine *di*phosphate (ADP).
2. When the ATP converts to ADP, the ATP is said to be *spent*.
3. Then the ADP is usually immediately recycled in the mitochondria where it is recharged and comes out again as ATP.

Functions of ATP (Fig. 8.5)

Respiration is the important process of all the living being, where oxygen is utilised and carbon dioxide is released from the body. During this process, energy is released, which is used to perform various functions of the body.

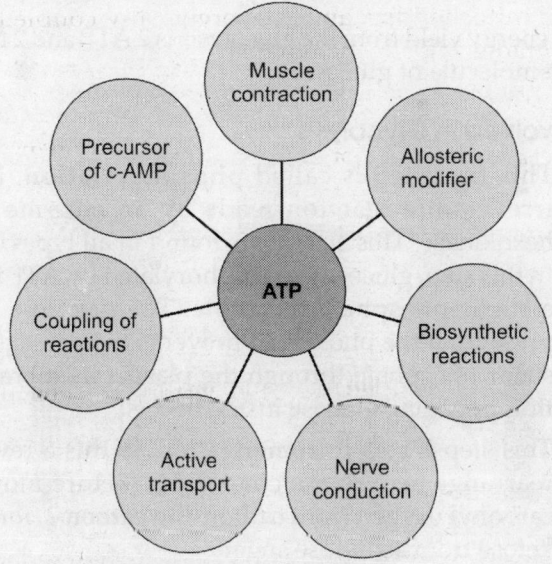

Fig. 8.5: Functions of ATP

In the provided content we will discuss two important mechanisms of respiration which are glycolysis and Krebs cycle.

GLYCOLYSIS AND KREBS CYCLE

Glycolysis is **defined** as the chain of the reactions, for the conversion of glucose (or glycogen) into pyruvate lactate and thus producing ATP. On the other hand, Krebs cycle or citric acid cycle **involves** the oxidation of acetyl CoA into CO_2 and H_2O.

Glycolysis is also known as 'Embden-Meyerhof-Parnas pathway'. It is a unique pathway occurring aerobically as well anaerobically, without the involvement of molecular oxygen. It is the major pathway for glucose metabolism and occurs in the cytoplasm of cells. The basic concept of this process is that the one molecule of glucose gets partially oxidized into two moles of pyruvate, enhanced by the presence of enzymes.

GLYCOLYSIS PATHWAY

Thus the energy yield from the glycolysis is 2 ATP and 2 NADH, from one molecule of glucose.

Steps Involved in Glycolysis

Step 1: This first step is called **phosphorylation**, it is an irreversible reaction leads by an enzyme called hexokinase. This enzyme is found in all types of cells. In this step, glucose is phosphorylated by ATP to form a sugar-phosphate molecule. The negative charge present on the phosphate prevents the passage of the sugar phosphate through the plasma membrane and thus engaging glucose inside the cell.

Step 2: This step is called **isomerization**, in this a reversible rearrangement of the chemical structure moves the carbonyl oxygen from carbon 1 to carbon 2, forming a ketose from an aldose sugar.

Step 3: This is also a **phosphorylation** step, the new hydroxyl group on carbon 1 is phosphorylated by ATP, for the formation of two to three carbon sugar phosphates. This step is regulated by the enzyme phospho-fructokinase, which checks the entry of sugars into glycolysis.

Flow chart 8.1: Glycolysis pathway

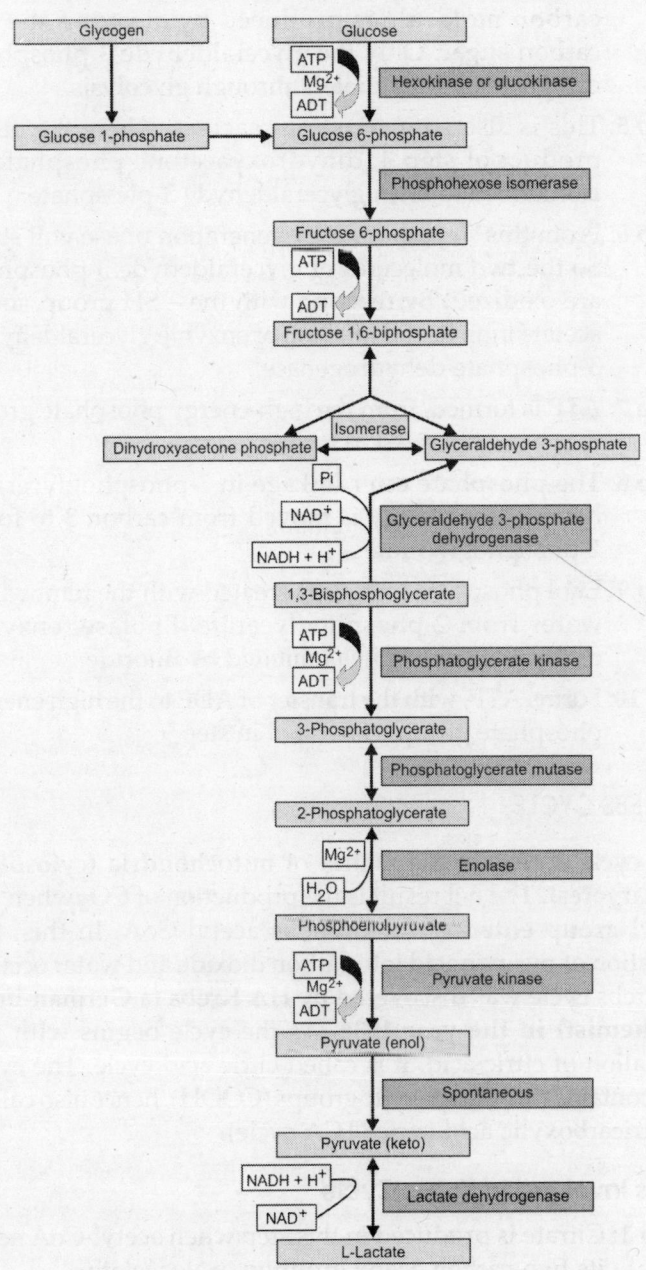

Step 4: This is named **cleavage reaction**. Here two three-carbon molecule is produced by cleaving the six carbon sugar. Only the glyceraldehyde 3-phosphate can proceed immediately through glycolysis.

Step 5: This is also **isomerization** reaction, where the other product of step 4, dihydroxyacetone phosphate is isomerized to form glyceraldehyde 3-phosphate.

Step 6: From this step, the energy generation phase will start. So the two molecules of glyceraldehyde 3-phosphate are oxidized. By reacting with the – SH group, iodo-acetate inhibits the function of enzyme glyceraldehyde-3-phosphate dehydrogenase.

Step 7: ATP is formed, from the high-energy phosphate group that was generated in step 6.

Step 8: The phosphate ester linkage in 3-phosphoglycerate, having free energy is moved from carbon 3 to form 2-phosphoglycerate.

Step 9: Enol phosphate linkage is created with the removal of water from 2-phosphoglycerate. Enolase (enzyme catalyzing this step) is inhibited by fluoride.

Step 10: Forms ATP, with the transfer of ADP to the high energy phosphate group, generated in step 9.

KREBS CYCLE

This cycle occurs in the matrix of **mitochondria (cytosol in prokaryotes)**. The net result is the production of CO_2 when the acetyl group entering the cycle as acetyl-CoA. In this, the oxidation of pyruvic acid into carbon dioxide and water occurs.

Krebs cycle was discovered by **HA Krebs (a German-born biochemist) in the year 1936**. As the cycle begins with the formation of citric acid, it is called citric acid cycle. The cycle also contains three carboxylic groups (COOH), hence also called as a tricarboxylic acid cycle (TCA cycle).

Steps Involved in Krebs Cycle

Step 1: Citrate is produced in this step when acetyl-CoA adds its two-carbon acetyl group to oxaloacetate.

Flow chart 8.2: The citric acid (Krebs) cycle

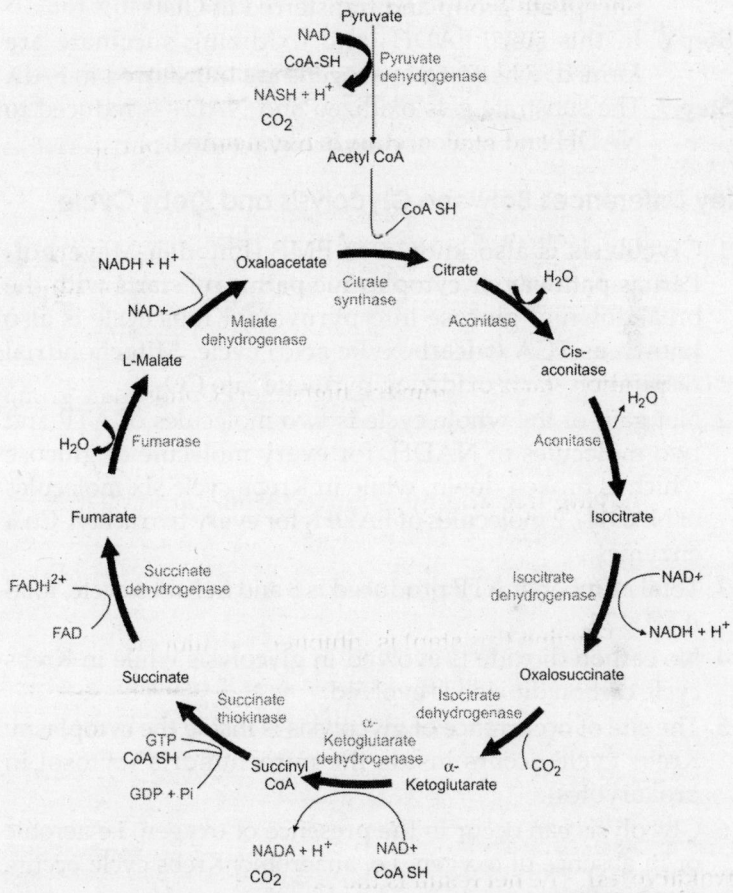

Step 2: Citrate is converted to its isocitrate (an isomer of citrate), by the removal of one water molecule and adding the another.

Step 3: NAD⁺ is reduced to NA when isocitrate is oxidized and loses a CO_2 molecule.

Step 4: CO_2 is lost again, the resulting compound is oxidized and NAD⁺ is reduced to NADH. The remaining molecule gets attached to coenzyme A through an unstable bond. Alpha-ketoglutarate dehydrogenase catalyzes the reaction.

Step 5: GTP is generated by the displacement of CoA by a phosphate group and transferred to GDP.

Step 6: In this step, $FADH_2$ and oxidizing succinate are formed, when two hydrogens are transferred to FAD.

Step 7: The substrate gets oxidized and NAD+ is reduced to NADH and oxaloacetate is regenerated.

Key Differences Between Glycolysis and Krebs Cycle

1. Glycolysis is also known as EMP (Embden-Meyerhof-Parnas pathway or cytoplasmic pathway) starts with the breakdown of glucose into pyruvate; Krebs cycle is also known as TCA (tricarboxylic acid) cycle. Mitochondrial respiration starts oxidizing pyruvate into CO_2.

2. Net gain of the whole cycle is two molecules of ATP and two molecules of NADH, for every molecule of glucose which is broken down, while in Krebs cycle six molecules of $NADH_2$, 2 molecules of $FADH_2$ for every two acetyl-CoA enzymes.

3. Total number of ATP produced is 8 and in Krebs cycle, total ATP is 24.

4. No carbon dioxide is evolved in glycolysis while in Krebs cycle carbon dioxide is evolved.

5. The site of occurrence of glycolysis is inside the cytoplasm; Krebs cycle occurs inside the mitochondria (cytosol in prokaryotes).

6. Glycolysis can occur in the presence of oxygen, i.e aerobic or in absence of oxygen, i.e. anaerobic; Krebs cycle occurs aerobically.

7. A glucose molecule is degraded into two molecules of an organic substance, pyruvate in glycolysis, while degradation of pyruvate is completely into inorganic substances which are CO_2 and H_2O.

8. In glycolysis 2 ATP molecules are consumed for the phosphorylation while Krebs cycle there is no consumption of ATP.

9. No role of oxidative phosphorylation in glycolysis; there is a major role of oxidative phosphorylation as well as oxaloacetate is considered to play a catalytic role in Krebs cycle.

10. As in glycolysis, glucose is broken into pyruvate, and hence glycolysis is said as the first step of respiration; Krebs cycle is the second step of respiration for the production of ATP.

11. Glycolysis is a straight or linear pathway; while Krebs cycle is a circular pathway.

Conclusion

Both the pathways produce energy for the cell, where glycolysis is the breakdown of a molecule of glucose to yield two molecules of pyruvate, whereas Krebs cycle is the process where acetyl-CoA produces citrate by adding its carbon acetyl group to oxaloacetate. Glycolysis is essential for the brain which depends on glucose for energy.

Krebs cycle is an important metabolic pathway in supplying energy to the body, about 65–70% of the ATP is synthesized in Krebs cycle. Citric acid cycle or Krebs cycle is the final oxidative pathway which connects almost all the individual metabolic pathway.

PHOTOSYNTHESIS

Photosynthesis is the process by which plants, some bacteria, and some protistans use the energy from sunlight to produce sugar, which cellular respiration converts into ATP, the "fuel" used by all living things. The conversion of unusable sunlight energy into usable chemical energy, is associated with the actions of the green pigment chlorophyll. Most of the time, the photosynthetic process uses water and releases the oxygen that we absolutely must have to stay alive. The overall reaction of this process is (Fig. 8.6)

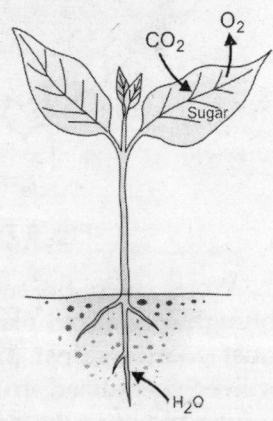

Fig. 8.6: Diagram of a typical plant, showing the inputs and outputs of the photosynthetic process

$$6H_2O + 6CO_2 \longrightarrow C_6H_{12}O_6 + 6O_2$$

LEAVES AND LEAF STRUCTURE

Plants are the only photosynthetic organisms to have leaves (and not all plants have leaves). A leaf may be viewed as a solar collector crammed full of photosynthetic cells.

The raw materials of photosynthesis, water and carbon dioxide, enter the cells of the leaf, and the products of photosynthesis, sugar and oxygen, leave the leaf (Fig. 8.7).

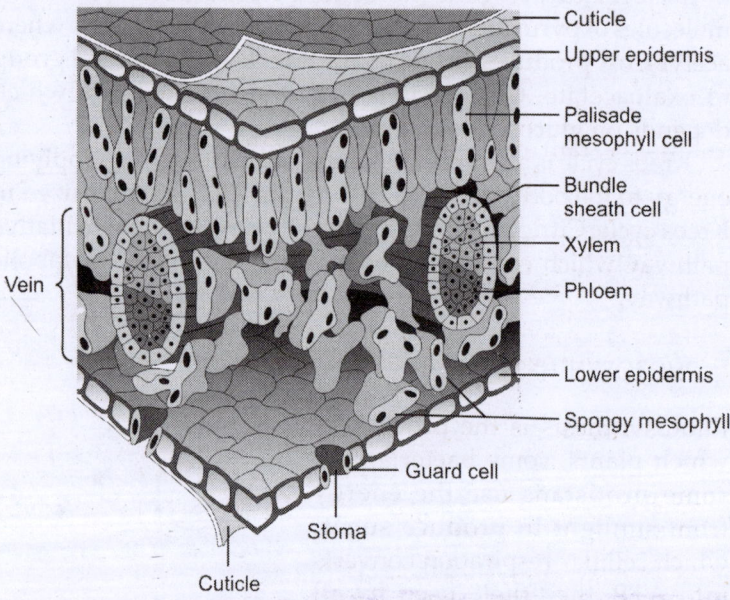

Fig. 8.7: Cross section of a leaf

Water enters the root and is transported up to the leaves through specialized plant cells known as xylem. Land plants must guard against drying out (desiccation) and so have evolved specialized structures known as stomata to allow gas to enter and leave the leaf. Carbon dioxide cannot pass through the protective waxy layer covering the leaf (cuticle), but it can enter the leaf through an opening (the stoma; plural = stomata; Greek for hole) flanked by two guard cells. Likewise, oxygen produced during photosynthesis can only pass out of the leaf through the opened stomata. Unfortunately for the plant, while these gases are moving between the inside and outside of the leaf, a great deal of water is also lost.

CHLOROPHYLL AND ACCESSORY PIGMENTS

A pigment is any substance that absorbs light. The color of the pigment comes from the wavelengths of light reflected (in other words, those not absorbed). Chlorophyll, the green pigment common to all photosynthetic cells, absorbs all wavelengths of visible light except green. Chlorophyll is a complex molecule. Several modifications of chlorophyll occur among plants and other photosynthetic organisms. All photosynthetic organisms (plants, certain protistans, prochlorobacteria, and cyanobacteria) have chlorophyll a. Accessory pigments absorb energy that chlorophyll a does not absorb. Accessory pigments include chlorophyll b (also c, d, and e in algae and protistans), xanthophylls, and carotenoids (such as beta-carotene). Chlorophyll a absorbs its energy from the violet-blue and reddish orange-red wavelengths, and little from the intermediate (green-yellow-orange) wavelengths.

Carotenoids and chlorophyll b absorb some of the energy in the green wavelength. Both chlorophylls also absorb in the orange-red end of the spectrum (with longer wavelengths and lower energy).

The Structure of the Chloroplast and Photosynthetic Membranes

The thylakoid is the structural unit of photosynthesis. Both photosynthetic prokaryotes and eukaryotes have these flattened sacs/vesicles containing photosynthetic chemicals. Only eukaryotes have chloroplasts with a surrounding membrane.

Thylakoids are stacked like pancakes in stacks known collectively as grana. The areas between grana are referred to as stroma. While the mitochondrion has two membrane systems, the chloroplast has three, forming three compartments (Fig. 8.8).

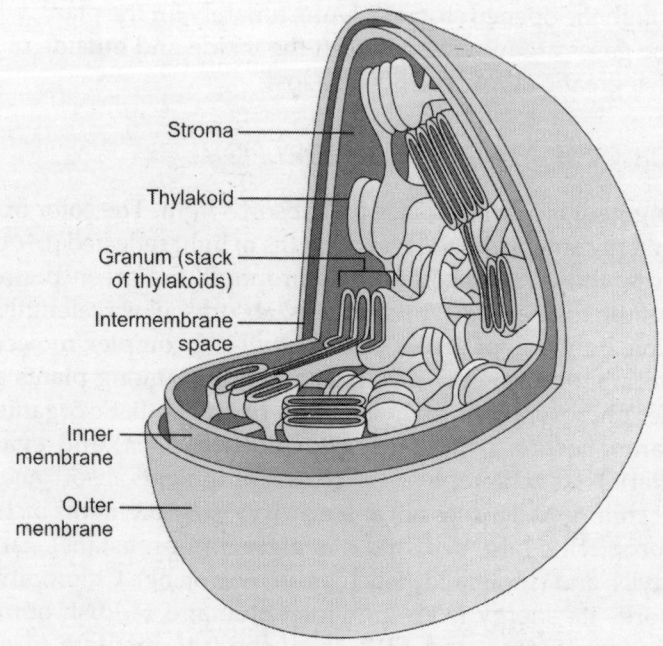

Fig. 8.8: Structure of chloroplast

STAGES OF PHOTOSYNTHESIS

Photosynthesis is a two-stage process.

The first process is the light-dependent process (light reactions) requires the direct energy of light to make energy carrier molecules that are used in the second process. It occurs in grana.

The light-independent process (or dark reactions) occurs when the products of the light reaction are used to form C-C covalent bonds of carbohydrates. The dark reactions can usually occur in the dark, if the energy carriers from the light process are present. Recent evidence suggests that a major enzyme of the dark reaction is indirectly stimulated by light, thus the term dark reaction is somewhat of a misnomer. Dark reactions take place in the stroma of the chloroplasts.

Light-Dependent Reactions

The first part of the process happens in the thylakoids of the chloroplasts and is the "light- dependent" reactions: The photosystems I and II absorb the photons from the sunlight and process them through the membranes of the thylakoids simultaneously. The photons excite electrons in the chlorophyll which then move through the electron transport chain and causes $NADP^-$ to combine with H^+ forming NADPH. At the same time, ADP (adenosine diphosphate) has come from the dark reaction and a third phosphate chain is bonded forming ATP (adenosine triphosphate) to feed the Calvin Cycle next. Remember that ATP is the important source of all cellular energy. Oxygen released in photosynthesis comes from the water molecules and all oxygen atoms that form the carbohydrates come from the carbon dioxide molecules. So, in other words, during the light-dependent reaction a water molecule is broken down producing two H^+ ions and a half an oxygen molecule. We get the rest of the oxygen molecule when another water molecule is broken down.

Dark Reactions

Dark reactions are also known as the Calvin Cycle, the Calvin-Benson cycle, and light-independent reactions. The point is that they do not require sunlight to complete their process. After ATP is formed in the first part of photosynthesis, for living things to grow, reproduce and repair themselves, the inorganic form of CO_2 must be transformed into carbohydrate. This happens during the Calvin Cycle in the stroma (the fluid filled interior of the chloroplast). ATP and NADPH combine with CO_2 and water to make the end product of glucose. The ADP and $NADPH^+$ are recycled to the light-dependent side.

Energy Yielding and Energy Consuming Reactions

Metabolism is a biochemical process that allows an organism to live, grow, reproduce, heal, and adapt to its environment. Anabolism and catabolism are two metabolic processes or phases. Anabolism refers to the process which builds molecules the body needs; it usually requires energy for completion.

Catabolism refers to the process that breaks down complex molecules into smaller molecules; it usually releases energy for the organism to use.

ANABOLIC AND CATABOLIC PROCESSES

Anabolic processes use simple molecules within the organism to create more complex and specialized compounds. In this synthesis, the creation of a product from a series of components, that is why anabolism is also called "biosynthesis." The process uses energy to create its end products, which the organism can use to sustain itself, grow, heal, reproduce or adjust to changes in its environment. Growing in height and muscle mass are two basic anabolic processes. At the cellular level, anabolic processes can use small molecules called monomers to build polymers, resulting in often highly complex molecules. For example, amino acids (monomers) can be synthesized into proteins (polymers), much like a builder can use bricks to create a large variety of buildings.

Catabolic processes break down complex compounds and molecules to release energy. This creates the metabolic cycle, where anabolism then creates other molecules that catabolism breaks down, many of which remain in the organism to be used again.

The principal catabolic process is digestion, where nutrient substances are ingested and broken down into simpler components for the body to use. In cells, catabolic processes break down polysaccharides such as starch, glycogen, and cellulose into monosaccharides (glucose, ribose and fructose, for example) for energy. Proteins are broken down into amino acids, for use in anabolic synthesis of new compounds or for recycling. And nucleic acids, found in RNA and DNA, are catabolized into nucleotides as part of the body's energy needs or for the purpose of healing (Table 8.2).

CONCEPT OF ENERGY CHARGE

The adenylate energy charge is an index used to measure the energy status of biological cells.

Table 8.2 Anabolism versus catabolism comparison chart

	Anabolic	Catabolic
Introduction	Metabolic process that builds molecules the body needs.	Metabolic process that breaks down large molecules into smaller molecules.
Energy	Requires energy	Releases energy
Hormones	Estrogen, testosterone, insulin, growth hormone.	Adrenaline, cortisol, glucagon, cytokines.
Effects on Exercise	Anabolic exercises, which are often anaerobic in nature, generally build muscle mass.	Catabolic exercises are usually aerobic and good at burning fat and calories.
Example	Amino acids becoming polypeptides (proteins), glucose becoming glycogen, fatty acids becoming triglycerides.	Proteins becoming amino acids, proteins becoming glucose, glycogen becoming glucose, or triglycerides becoming fatty acids.

ATP or Mg-ATP is the principal molecule for storing and transferring energy in the cell. It is used for biosynthetic pathways, maintenance of transmembrane gradients, movement, cell division, etc. More than 90% of the ATP is produced by phosphorylation of ADP by the ATP synthase. ATP can also be produced by "substrate level phosphorylation" reactions (ADP phosphorylation by (1,3)-bisphosphoglycerate, phosphoenolpyruvate, phosphocreatine), by the succinate-CoA ligase and phosphoenolpyruvate carboxylkinase, and by adenylate kinase, an enzyme that maintains the three adenine nucleotides in equilibrium.

The energy charge is related to ATP, ADP and AMP concentrations. It was first defined by Atkinson and Walton who found that it was necessary to take into account the concentration of all three nucleotides, rather than just ATP and ADP, to account for the energy status in metabolism. Since the adenylate kinase maintains two ADP molecules in equilibrium with one ATP, Atkinson defined the adenylate energy charge as:

$$\text{Energy charge} = \frac{[ATP] + 1/2\,[ADP]}{[ATP] + [ADP] + [AMP]}$$

The energy charge of most cells varies between 0.75 and 0.90. Life depends on an adequate energy charge. If ATP synthesis is momentarily insufficient to maintain an adequate energy charge, AMP can be converted by two different pathways to uric acid. This helps to buffer the adenylate energy charge by decreasing the total [ATP + ADP + AMP] concentration.

KEY POINTS

- The First Law of Thermodynamics, also known as the law of conservation of energy, states that energy can neither be created nor destroyed.
- The Second Law of Thermodynamics states that when energy is transferred, there will be less energy available at the end of the transfer process than at the beginning.
- Exothermic reactions may occur spontaneously and result in higher randomness or entropy ($\Delta S > 0$) of the system and decrease in enthalpy ($\Delta H < 0$).
- Endothermic reactions are characterized by positive heat flow (into the reaction) and an increase in enthalpy ($+\Delta H$). Example is photosynthesis.
- The nucleotide coenzyme adenosine triphosphate (ATP) is the most important form of chemical energy in all cells.
- ATP is a nucleoside triphosphate containing adenine, ribose, and three phosphate groups.
- There are two basic mechanisms involved for ATP formation:
  1. Substrate level phosphorylation and
  2. Oxidative phosphorylation
- Substrate level phosphorylation—involves phosphorylation of ADP to form ATP at the expense of the energy of the parent substrate molecule without involving the electron transport chain.
- ATP by oxidative phosphorylation—this process takes place in mitochondria and is energetically coupled to a proton gradient over a membrane.
- **Respiration** is the important process of all the living beings, where oxygen is utilised and carbon dioxide is released from the body.

- Glycolysis is **defined** as the chain of the reactions, for the conversion of glucose (or glycogen) into pyruvate lactate and thus producing ATP.
- Krebs cycle or citric acid cycle **involves** the oxidation of acetyl-CoA into CO_2 and H_2O.
- Krebs cycle: This cycle occurs in the matrix of mitochondria (cytosol in prokaryotes).
- Krebs cycle was discovered by **HA Krebs (a German-born biochemist) in the year 1936.** As the cycle begins with the formation of citric acid, it is called citric acid cycle.
- Photosynthesis is the process by which plants, some bacteria, and some protistans use the energy from sunlight to produce sugar, which cellular respiration converts into ATP.
- Stages of photosynthesis:
  1. The first process is the light-dependent Process (light reactions), requires the direct energy of light to make energy carrier molecules—occurs in grana.
  2. The light-independent process (or dark reactions). The dark reactions can usually occur in the dark—occur in the stroma of the chloroplasts.
- Anabolic processes use simple molecules within the organism to create more complex and specialized compounds—this is why anabolism is also called "biosynthesis".
- Catabolic processes break down complex compounds and molecules to release energy. The principal catabolic process is digestion, where nutrient substances are ingested and broken down into simpler components for the body to use.

PRACTICE QUESTIONS

Very Short Answer Type Questions

1. What is the primary source of energy for living organisms?
2. Give one biological example of (a) endothermic reaction, (b) exothermic reaction.
3. What is spontaneous reaction?
4. Give full form of: (a) ATP, (b) EMP, (c) NADH.

5. What is the site of occurrence of glycolysis?
6. How many ATP are produced in glycolysis?
7. What is the structural unit of photosynthesis?
8. What are the two stages in photosynthesis?
9. What is anabolism?
10. Give the full form of: (a) ADP, (b) NADPH.

Short Answer Type Questions

1. Explain the first law of thermodynamics in biological systems.
2. Give differences between: (a) Exothermic and endothermic reactions, (b) Endergonic and exergonic reactions.
3. Give the relation of K_{eq} with standard free energy.
4. Define glycolysis.
5. What is the role of chlorophyll in photosynthesis.

Long Answer Type Questions

1. Explain how ATP is produced.
2. Explain the process of glycolysis.
3. Give differences between glycolysis and Krebs cycle.
4. Explain the two stages of photosynthesis.
5. What is energy charge?
6. Give differences between anabolism and catabolism.

Microbiology

INTRODUCTION OF MICROBIOLOGY

The field of microbiology has traditionally been concerned with information on how cells respond to their environment, interact with each other, or undergo complex processes such as cellular differentiation or gene expression.

"Microbiology is the study of all organisms that are invisible to the naked eye, that is the study of micro-organisms, i.e. viruses, bacteria, many algae and fungi, and protozoa."

Micro-organisms are necessary for the production of bread, cheese, beer, antibiotics, vaccines, vitamins, enzymes, etc. Modern **biotechnology** rests upon a microbiological foundation.

CONCEPT OF SINGLE CELLED ORGANISMS

What is Living Organism?

A life form capable of growing and reproducing by itself is known as living organism. The main characteristics of life include the following:

161

1. **Responsiveness** to the environment
2. **Growth**
3. Ability to **reproduce**
4. Cellular organization
5. Ability to perform **metabolism**
6. Maintain **homeostasis**
7. Passing traits onto offspring.

Out of the above most defining characters of living organisms are:

1. **Responsiveness** to the environment
2. Ability to perform **metabolism**
3. Cellular organization

Viruses are not classified as living organisms on the basis of their nucleic acid content because they cannot survive in their own.

Classification of Organisms

Living organism can be unicellular or multicellular (Table 9.1).

Table 9.1 Comparison between unicellular and multicellular

Unicellular organisms	Multicellular organisms
The body of the organism is composed of single cell	The body of the organism is composed of numerous cell
Prokaryotic in nature	Eukaryotic in nature.
Vegetative/asexual reproduction	Sexual type of reproduction
A single cell carries out all life processes	Different cells are specialized to perform different functions
Injury of the cell can cause death of the organism	Injury or death of some cells does not affect the organism as the same can be replaced by new ones.
Some examples of a unicellular animal are Amoebae, slime mould, algae, malaria parasite	Humans are multicellular

Single Cell Concept

In the field of cellular biology, **single cell analysis** is the study of genomics, transcriptomics, proteomics and metabolomics at the single cell level. *In situ* sequencing and fluorescence *in situ* hybridization (FISH) do not require that cells be isolated and are increasingly being used for analysis of tissues (Fig. 9.1) (Table 9.2).

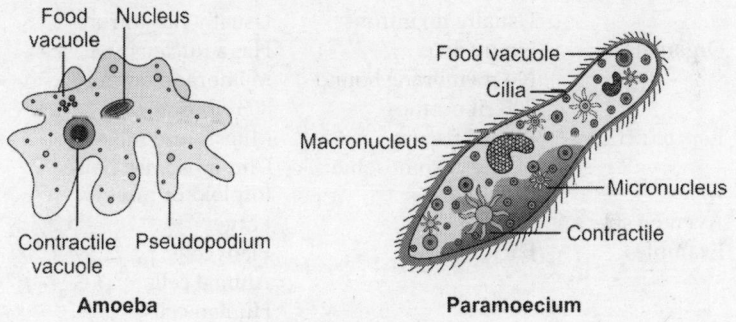

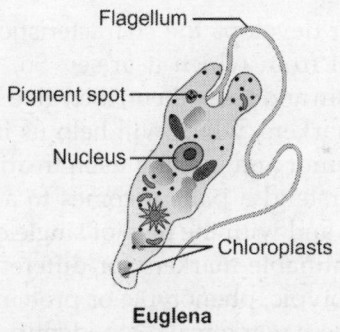

Fig. 9.1: Unicellular organisms

Single Cell Concept and Analysis

Multicellular organisms studied in group of cells, tissues organs and body give information which is not completely informative because individual cells of different parts of body of multi-cellular organism are not represented in these assays.

To overcome this obstacle the concept of single cell isolation from multicellular organisms and studying their structure and metabolic pathways and genomic expressions have been developed.

For example, human brain is made up of many type of cells like oligodendrocytes, astrocytes, etc.

Table 9.2 Classification of organism based on cell structure

	Prokaryotes	Eukaryotes
DNA	DNA is naked	DNA bound to protein
	DNA is circular	DNA is linear
	Usually no introns	Usually has introns
Organelles	No nucleus	Has a nucleus
	No membrane bound	Membrane-bound
	70S ribosomes	80S ribosomes
Reproduction	Binary fission	Mitosis and meiosis
	Single chromosome (haploid)	Chromosomes paired (diploid or more)
Average size	Smaller	Larger
Examples	Bacteria cells	Plant cells
		Animal cells
		Human cells

If a brain tumor develops the characteristic of that tumor will match the cell from which it arises. So, we isolate the different cells of brain and assay them, then give specific protein markers or gene markers, which will help us in knowing the pathology of the tumor and helping us in treating that tumor.

Now you understand a patient comes to a neurosurgeon with a brain tumor and with the help of single cell concept we have different identifiable markers for different type of cells which may be genotypic, phenotypic or proteinecious.

Now through these markers we can identify the tumor and develop a particular type of treatment for it.

So, single cell concept of living organisms for study was developed (Fig. 9.2).

Single Cell Isolation

Many single cell analysis techniques require the isolation of individual cells. Methods currently used for single cell isolation include serial dilution, micromanipulation, laser capture microdissection, FACS, microfluidics, manual picking, enzymatic digestion, and Raman tweezers.

Manual single cell picking is a method where cells in a suspension are viewed under a microscope, and individually picked using a micropipette.

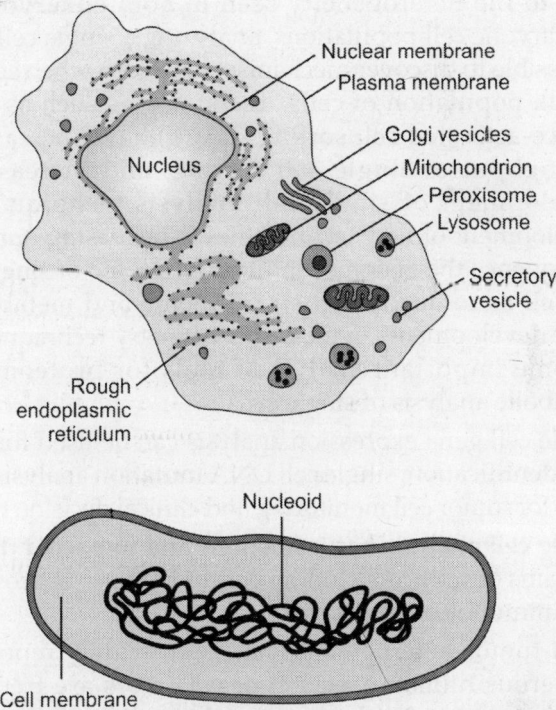

Fig. 9.2: Cell of prokaryotic and eukaryotic cell structure

Raman tweezers is a technique where Raman spectroscopy is combined with optical tweezers, which uses a laser beam to trap, and manipulate cells.

Benefits of Single Cell Concept

1. In conventional based assays heterogeneity of individual cells is ignored.
2. Cell to cell differences in RNA transcript and protein expression are ignored.
3. To better understand the variations from cell to cell, scientists need to use single cell analyses to provide more detailed information for therapeutic decision making in precision medicine.

4. Due to the heterogeneity seen in both eukaryotic and prokaryotic cell populations, analyzing a single cell makes it possible to discover mechanisms not seen when studying a bulk population of cells. Technologies such as fluorescence-activated cell sorting (FACS) have increased the throughput of single cell sorting, and increased the development of single cell analysis techniques. The development of new technologies is increasing our ability to sequence the genome, and transcriptome of single cells, as well as to quantify their proteome and metabolome. New developments in mass spectrometry techniques have become important analytical tools for proteomic and metabolic analysis of single cells.

5. Single cell gene expression analysis can be used for tumor cell identification; single cell DNA mutation analysis can be used for tumor cell monitoring and clinical decision making.

6. Single cell analysis has influenced and impacted different domains of science including cancer biology, neuroscience, and immunology and so on.

7. Intra-tumor heterogeneity has been widely reported in numerous human cancer types. Tumors are frequently composed of individual, molecularly distinct clones that differ in their proliferation rates and metastatic potential, most critically, in their sensitivities and responses to drug treatment. Those cells that can cause distant metastases should possess unique characteristics when compared to the remaining subpopulation.

8. Stem cells are undifferentiated cells that are characterized as both being capable of self-renewal and having the potential to differentiate into specialized types of cells. How stem cells balance their self-renewal capacity and their ability to differentiate are central questions in stem cell research.

CONCEPT OF SPECIES AND STRAINS

A **species** is a class of plants or animals whose members have the same main characteristics and are able to breed with each other. The species could be described as 'a genomically coherent cluster of individual organisms that show a high degree of overall similarity in many independent characteristics and is diagnosable by a unique phenotypic property'.

A **strain** is a low-level taxonomic rank used at the intraspecific level (within a species). Strains are often seen as inherently artificial concepts, characterized by a specific intent for genetic isolation. This is most easily observed in microbiology where strains are derived from a single cell colony and are typically quarantined by the physical constraints of a Petri dish.

Serotype: A serotype is a sub-group of species, which are grouped according to their antigenic properties. Antigens are substances that are considered "foreign" to the host body. The host combats these antigens by eliciting an immune response, which involves the production of antibodies. These antibodies are found in serum ('sero-'), which is a part of our circulatory system.

Thus, **serotypes** are sub-groups of the same species of micro-organism which share similar antigens (antigenically), and the antibodies that are directed against those antigens are the same (serologically).

IDENTIFICATION AND CLASSIFICATION OF MICRO-ORGANISMS

Basic Terms Used in Classification

1. **Phylogenetic classification system:** Groups reflect genetic similarity and evolutionary relatedness.
2. **Phenetic classification system:** Groups do not necessarily reflect genetic similarity or evolutionary relatedness. Instead, groups are based on convenient, observable characteristics.
3. **Taxonomy:** Taxonomy, in a broad sense the science of classification, but more strictly the classification of living and extinct organisms—i.e. biological classification. The term is derived from the Greek *taxis* ("arrangement") and *nomos* ("law").

4. **Species:** A collection of microbial strains that share many properties and differ significantly from other groups of strains.

5. **Strain:** A population of organisms descended from a single organism or pure culture isolate.

6. **Systematics** refers to the study and classification of organisms for the determination of the evolutionary relationship of organisms. Therefore, the systematics consists of both taxonomy and evolution. Systematics uses morphological, behavioral, genetics, and evolutionary relationships between organisms.

7. **Morphology** is the study of how things are put together, like the make-up of animals and plants, or the branch of linguistics that studies the structure of words. In **morphology**, the word part *morph-* **means** "form" and *-ology* "the study of".

8. **Vertical genetic transfer** occurs when there is gene exchange from the parental generation to the offspring.

9. **Lateral/ horizontal genetic transfer (LGT)** is then a mechanism of gene exchange that happens independently of reproduction.

Micro-organisms

Micro-organisms are everywhere; almost every natural surface is colonized by microbes, from body to ocean. A suitable standard for measuring microbes is the micrometer which is six times smaller than a meter (one-millionth of a meter). There are 10^6 µm in **one meter**, and it is these units that are used to measure the size of bacteria. Typically, bacteria range from about 1 µm to about 5 µm. **Antony van Leewenhoek** (1632–1723) who invented the first microscope (50–300x) and was the first to accurately observe and describe micro-organisms. Living organism (such as bacteria too small to be seen with naked eye but visible under a microscope. They are also called microbes. Micro-organisms are very diverse. They include bacteria, fungi, algae, and protozoa; microscopic plants, and animals.

Goals of Classification

To identify different species of living organisms into an hierarchical pattern based on multiple criteria like morphology, structure, metabolic activities genome and genetic associations.

Reasons for Classification

1. Same species have different names in different languages in different regions of the earth.
2. To create a uniformity by creating a nomenclature on the basis of classification in scientific terms, so that same species have same name in all scientific field of study.
3. To evaluate any changes in the characters of species like creation of strains, subspecies, serotypes can be properly recorded.
4. Easy identification of the unknown species.

Methods of Identification of Micro-organism

1. Phenotypic method
2. Phylogenetic method
3. Other methods
   a. Numerical taxonomy
   b. DNA homology
   c. Ribosomal RNA homology

Phenotypic Method

The organisms can be classified on the basis of cell structure, cellular metabolism, or on differences in cell components. Classification seeks to describe the diversity of bacterial species by naming and grouping organisms based on similarities. Micro-organisms can be classified on the basis of cell structure, cellular metabolism, or on differences in cell components such as DNA, fatty acids, pigments, and antigens.

Phylogenetic Method

Phylogenetic analysis is to understand the past evolutionary path of organisms. Due to technological innovation in modern molecular biology and the rapid advancement in computational science, accurate inference of the phylogeny of a gene or organism seems possible in the near future.

Other Methods

1. **Numerical taxonomy:** Based on their characteristic states using numerical algorithms rather than using subjective evaluation of their properties.

   Process: Many characteristics of an organism are studied (usually 100–200) and each characteristic is given equal weight. Then the percent similarity is calculated. They are often summarized with a treelike diagram called "Dendrogram".

   Advantages:
   a. Relatively unbiased.
   b. Greater degree of stability and predictability.

   Disadvantages:
   a. Only useful within larger groups.
   b. Exclusively depends upon the mathematical figures plotted on the paper.
   c. Cannot be related to any particular taxonomic group such as genus or species.

2. **DNA homology:** Double stranded DNA molecules from two different organisms are heated to convert them to single strands. Mixed those single strands and allowed to cool. If the two organisms are closely related hetero duplexes (a strand from one organism will pair with a strand from the other organism)

3. **Ribosomal RNA homology:** Ribosomes as a chronometer of evolution and tool for determining genetic relatedness.

   Advantages:
   a. 16S rRNA gene is present in all bacteria.
   b. Large subunit (LSU) gene is present in all fungi.
   c. Identical in all micro-organisms.
   d. Different in many micro-organisms.
   e. High content of information

Disadvantages

a. Expensive.

b. PCR bias may happened

All methods are very useful in terms of classification of micro-organism but DNA homology and rRNA homology technologies are at the top because of their high stability and predictability.

Viruses

Similar to the classification systems used for cellular organisms, virus classification is the subject of ongoing debate due to their pseudo-living nature. Essentially, they are non-living particles with some chemical characteristics similar to those of life; but they do not have nucleus and cannot sustain independently and they require a host to carry out their biological activities. They are mostly pathogenic to animals and plants causing various diseases like human immunodeficiency virus (HIV), herpesvirus, etc.

Viruses are mainly classified by phenotypic characteristics, such as:

1. Morphology
2. Nucleic acid type
3. Mode of replication
4. Host organisms
5. Type of disease they cause

MICROSCOPY

The microscope, is an instrument that produces enlarged images of small objects, allowing the observer an exceedingly close view of minute structures.

Principles of Light Microscopy

Light passes through specimen and series of magnifying lenses. The important factors in light microscopy are:

1. **Magnification:**
   a. Simple microscope has one magnifying lens

b. Compound microscope has 2 magnifying lenses. It is most commonly used in educational labs (Fig. 9.3).
   i. Ocular lens
   ii. Objective lens

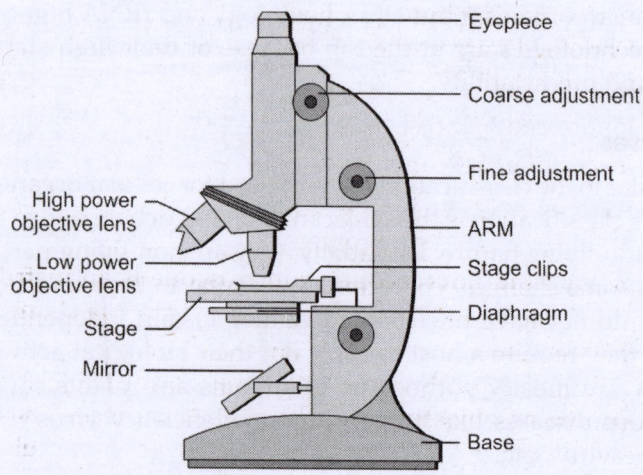

Fig. 9.3: A compound microscope with its various parts

Magnification is equal to the product of ocular lens and the objective lens, e.g.

$$10x \times 100x = 1000x$$

2. **Resolution:** Resolving power is defined as the minimum distance existing between two points where they still appear as separate.
   Resolving power determines how much detail can be seen:
   Naked eye = 0.1 mm
   Light microscope = 0.2 micrometer
   Electron microscope = 2.5 nm

3. **Contrast:** Reflects the number of visible shades in a specimen, it is done through staining of the specimen.

4. **Refractive index:** Refractive index is the light bending ability of a medium, the light may bend in air so much that it misses the small high-magnification lens, the refractive indexes of oil and glass are similar and immersion oil is used to keep light from bending.

TYPES OF MICROSCOPY

The eight types of microscopy are:

1. Compound microscope
2. Bright field microscopy
3. Dark field microscopy
4. Phase contrast microscopy
5. Fluorescent microscopy
6. Electron microscopy
7. Transmission electron microscopy
8. Scanning electron microscopy.

1. **Compound microscope:** A microscope is an instrument which makes enlarged image of minute objects near the objective lens.

   The compound microscope has two set lenses. One is known as objective and the other eyepiece. These are mounted in a holder commonly known as body tube. The lens system nearest to the specimen is called objective, while the second lens system is called eyepiece which is the nearest to eye.

2. **Bright field microscopy:** In bright field microscopy, the microscope field (the area observed) is bright and the micro-organisms appear dark because they absorb some of the light. Generally microscope of this type produces useful magnification of about X1000 to X2000.

3. **Dark field microscopy:** In this type of microscopy, a dark background is produced against which objects are brilliantly illuminated. Any object within this beam of light will reflect some light into the objective and will be visible. This method of illuminating an object where the object appears self-illuminous against a dark field, called dark-field illustration.

4. **Phase contrast microscopy:** The phase contrast principle was discovered by Fritz Zernike who was awarded Nobel Prize in physics in 1953. The phase contrast microscope is an ordinary bright field microscope with two additional plates, namely annular diaphragm and phase shifting plate,

which enables the usage forming rings to be phase shifted with respect to others. Annular diaphragm allows only a ray of light to pass through the condenser and then to object.

5. **Fluorescent microscopy:** Many chemical substances absorb light. After absorbing light of a particular wavelength and energy, some substances emit light of larger wavelength and lesser energy content.

   Such substances are called fluorescent and the phenomenon is termed fluorescence. This is the phenomenon which is applied in fluorescent microscopy. A high intensity mercury lamp is used as light source which emits white light.

6. **Electron microscopy:** In 1931 Knoll and Ruska, German scientists discovered electron microscopy. Von Borries and Ruska (1938) in Berlin constructed first practical electron microscope.

   In electron microscope the source of illumination is electron beam. The construction and principle of electron microscope are easily related to those of light microscope. The range of wavelength of visible light used in light microscope is 4000 Å–7800 Å, while with an electron microscope employing 60–80 kV electron, the wavelength is only 0.05 Å.

   In the instrument, the electron gun generates electron beam. These electrons are concentrated by other components of electron gun producing a fast moving narrow beam of electron.

   Electrons are focused by electromagnetic lenses. Electromagnetic lens consists of wire encased in soft iron casing. When electric current is passed through the coil, it generates an electromagnetic field through which electrons are focused.

7. **Transmission electron microscope:** The electron source is commonly a tungsten filament of 30–150 kV potential. The electron beam passes through the center of ring-like magnetic condenser and becomes converged on the specimen.

After being transmitted through the specimen [hence transmission electron microscope (TEM)], the magnetic objective focuses the electron into a first (real) image of the object which is enlarged (2000 times). The magnetic projector lens then magnifies a portion of the first image producing magnification up to 240,000 or more.

The final enlarged image can be reviewed by striking a fluorescent screen which makes it visible.

8. **Scanning Electron Microscopy (SEM):** Scanning electron microscopes combine the mechanism of electron microscopy and television. In SEM, electrons are not transmitted through the very thin specimen from below but impinge on its surface from above. The specimen may be opaque and of any manageable thickness and size.

Classification of Micro-organisms Based on Morphology

The micro-organisms can be classified and identified by their shapes (Fig. 9.4).

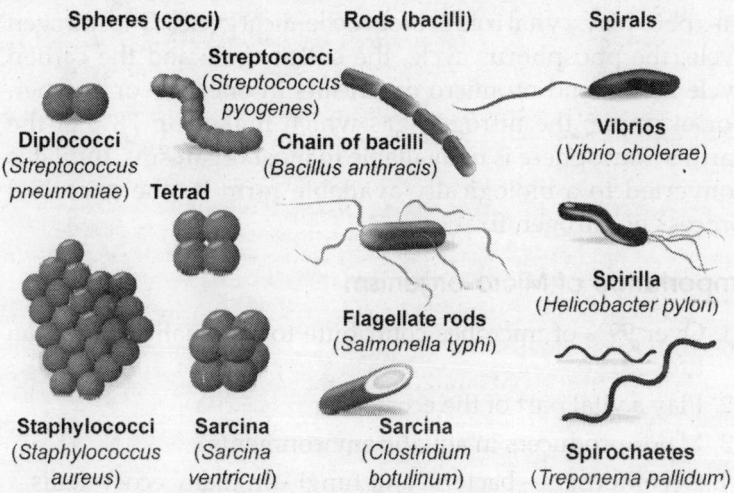

Fig. 9.4: Various types of bacteria based on their shapes

ECOLOGICAL ASPECTS OF MICRO-ORGANISM

Microbial Ecology

Micro-organisms, by their omnipresence, impact the entire biosphere. Microbial life plays a primary role in regulating biogeochemical systems in virtually all of our planet's environments, including some of the most extreme, from frozen environments and acidic lakes, to hydrothermal vents at the bottom of deepest oceans, and some of the most familiar, such as the human small intestine. Aside from carbon fixation, micro-organisms' key collective metabolic processes (including nitrogen fixation, methane metabolism, and sulfur metabolism) control global biogeochemical cycling.

Micro-organisms are the backbone of all ecosystems, but even more so in the zones where photosynthesis is unable to take place because of the absence of light. In such zones, chemo-synthetic microbes provide energy and carbon to the other organisms.

Other microbes are decomposers, with the ability to recycle nutrients from other organisms' waste products. These microbes play a vital role in biogeochemical cycles. The nitrogen cycle, the phosphorus cycle, the sulfur cycle and the carbon cycle all depend on micro-organisms in one way or another. For example, the nitrogen gas which makes up 78% of the earth's atmosphere is unavailable to most organisms, until it is converted to a biologically available form by the microbial process of nitrogen fixation.

Importance of Micro-organism

1. Over 99% of microbes contribute to the quality of human life
2. Play a vital part of the ecosystem
3. Major producers in aquatic environments
4. Decomposers—bacteria and fungi—in many ecosystems
5. Key role in biogeochemical cycles to recycle carbon, nitrogen, water

6. Natural pest killers in gardens and on crops
7. Serving as natural water treatment
8. Involved in many symbiotic relations as lichens, human digestion, rumens of cows

STERILIZATION AND MEDIA COMPOSITIONS

Sterilization

Sterilization is making a substance free from all micro organisms both in vegetative and sparing states. Spore is a reproductive structure that is adapted for dispersal and surviving for extended periods of time in unfavorable conditions. Spores form part of the lifecycles of many bacteria, plants, algae, fungi and some protozoa.

Terms Used in Sterilization

1. **Disinfection:** Disinfection does not affect spore state organisms. The destruction or removal of all pathogenic organisms capable of giving rise to infection.

2. **Antisepsis:** The term is used to indicate the prevention of infection, usually by inhibiting the growth of bacteria in wounds or tissues. This is done by the antiseptics, chemicals or disinfectants which can be safely applied on skin or mucous membrane to prevent infection by inhibiting the growth of bacteria like iodine.

3. **Bactericidal agents/germicides:** Those which able to kill bacteria

4. **Bacteriostatic agent:** Only prevent multiplication of bacteria, but they remain alive.

Cleaning

Important preparatory step before sterilization or disinfection, by removing soil and other dirt.

Decontamination

The process of rendering an article or area free of contaminants, including microbial, chemical, radioactive and other hazards.

Classification of Sterilization

1. Physical methods.
2. Chemical methods

Commonly Used Chemical for Sterilization

Alcohol

Frequently used are ethyl alcohol, isopropyl alcohol. These must be used at concentration 60–90%. Isopropyl alcohol is used in disinfection of clinical thermometer. Methyl alcohol is effective against fungal spores, treating cabinets and incubators. Methyl alcohol is also toxic and inflammable.

Aldehyde

Formaldehyde: Having bactericidal, sporicidal and has lethal effect on viruses. It is used to preserve anatomical specimens, destroying anthrax spores on hair and wool.

Glutaldehyde: Effective against tubercle bacilli, fungi, viruses. Less toxic and irritant to eyes, skin, it is used to treat anesthetic rubber, face masks, metal instruments and polythene tubing.

Gases

Types of gases used for sterilization:

1. Ethylene oxide
2. Beta propiolactone (BPL).

Formaldehyde Gas

This is widely employed for fumigation of OT and other rooms. Formaldehyde is produced by adding 150g of $KMnO_4$ to 280 ml of formalin for every 1000 cu.ft of room volume, after closing the windows and other outlets. After fumigation, the doors should be sealed and left unopened for 48 hours.

Chemical Indicators of Successful Sterilization

1. Tape with lines that change color when the intended temperature has been reached.
2. Indicator strips that show that the chemicals and/or gas are still effective.

3. Chemical indicators are available for testing ethylene oxide, dry heat, and steam processes. These indicators are used internally, placed where steam or temperature take longest to reach, or put on the outside of the wrapped packs to distinguish processed from no processed.
4. Bacterial culture results are needed before sterilization effectiveness can be determined.

Generally Used Sterilization Methods in Laboratory

1. **Dry heat:** Glassware and plasticware (empty vessels), and instruments may be sterilized by dry heat in an oven at 160–180°C for 3 hr. But most people prefer to autoclave. More recently, glass bead sterilizers (300°C) are being employed for the sterilization of forceps. These devices use dry heat.

2. **Flame sterilization:** Instruments like forceps, scalpels, needles, etc. are ordinarily flame sterilized by dipping them in 95% alcohol followed by flaming. These instruments are repeatedly sterilized during the operation to avoid contamination. It is customary to flame the mouths of culture vessels prior to inoculation/subculture.

3. **Autoclaving:** Culture vessels, etc. (both empty and containing media) are generally sterilized by heating in an autoclave or a pressure cooker to 121°C for 40 minutes. Sterilization during autoclaving depends mainly on temperature. Certain types of plasticware and some instrument, e.g. micropipettes, etc. are also autoclaved. Care should be taken to properly stopper all the vessels and to open the autoclave only when its pressure gauge indicates zero pressure.

Important Facts about Sterilization

1. Sterilization is a process or killing all micro-organisms (including spores) on or in a material or object.
2. The factors that determine the type of sterilization or disinfecting process to be used include time, temperature, stage of growth of the organism, nature of the medium in which the organism is suspended (air, gas, liquid) and the number of organism present.

3. Sterilization and disinfection can be achieved by using heat, filtration, chemical or radiation, etc.
4. Overall, heat is the best means of sterilization, but other methods are used for heat labile objects.
5. Dry heat requires more time than wet heat to kill organisms, boiling kills most vegetative cells but not bacterial spores and pressure cookers and autoclaves achieve sterilization.

Culture Medium

The food material or substances required for growing micro-organisms *in vitro* (outside the body) is called **culture medium**.

Types of Culture Media

Classification based on physical state:
1. Solid medium
2. Semi-solid medium
3. Liquid medium

Uses of Culture Medium

It is important to grow micro-organisms outside the body for the following purposes:
1. To identify the cause of infection from the clinical sample, so that proper treatment can be given.
2. To study the characteristics or properties of micro-organisms.
3. To prepare biological products like vaccines, toxoids, antigens, etc.

Composition of Culture Media

1. Water
2. Energy source
3. Carbon source
4. Nitrogen source
5. Mineral salts
6. Special growth factors

Classification Based on Physical State Solid Medium

Agar is the most commonly used solidifying agent. Agar is:

1. Golden-yellow granular powder
2. Prepared from seaweeds.
3. Not affected by the growth of the bacteria.
4. Melts at 98°C and sets at 42°C

Semi-solid Media

Such media are soft and are useful in demonstrating bacterial motility and separating motile from nonmotile strains. Liquid media are sometimes referred to as **"broth"**. Bacteria grow uniformly producing general turbidity, e.g. Nutrient broth.

Classification Based on the Ingredient

1. **Simple media:**
   - e.g.: Nutrient broth (NB).
   - NB consists of peptone, meat extract, NaCl.
   - NB + 2% agar = Nutrient agar
2. **Complex media:** Such as blood agar, it has ingredients that exact components are difficult to estimate.

Synthetic or Defined Media

Specially prepared media from pure chemical substances for research purpose and composition of every component is well known, e.g.: peptone water –1% peptone + 0.5% NaCl in water.

Special Media

1. Enriched media
2. Selective media
3. Differential media
4. Transport media
5. Anaerobic media

Enriched Media

1. Substances like blood, serum, egg are added to the simple medium.

2. Used to grow bacteria that are exacting in their nutritional needs, e.g.: Blood agar, chocolate agar.

Blood Agar

BAP contains mammalian blood (usually sheep or horse) typically at a concentration of 5–10%, used to isolate fastidious organisms and detect haemolysis.

Chocolate Agar

It contains red blood cells that have been lysed by slowly heating to 80°C and it is used for growing fastidious bacteria, such as *Haemophilus influenzae*.

GROWTH KINETICS

What is Microbial Growth?

Most micro-organisms divide and reproduce asexually. Binary fission and everything is equally divided between the two daughter cells (Fig. 9.5).

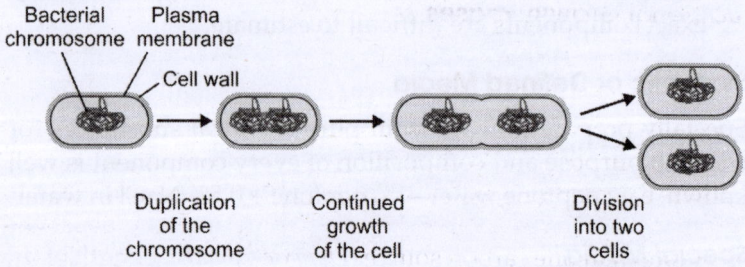

Bacterial   Plasma
chromosome   membrane

Cell wall

Duplication   Continued   Division
of the   growth   into two
chromosome   of the cell   cells

Fig. 9.5: Binary fission

Time it takes for a single cell to go from one division to the next is called **generation time** or **doubling time**. This is also the time it takes for a population to double. For many "typical" bacteria under "ideal" conditions, this doubling time may be as fast as 20 minutes.

Microbial **growth kinetics**: The relationship between the specific **growth** rate (μ) of a microbial population and the substrate concentration (s), is an indispensable tool in all fields of microbiology, be it physiology, genetics, ecology, or biotechnology.

Bacterial Growth Curve

When an organism is inoculated into a nutrient solution 4 distinct growth phases are noted (Fig. 9.6).

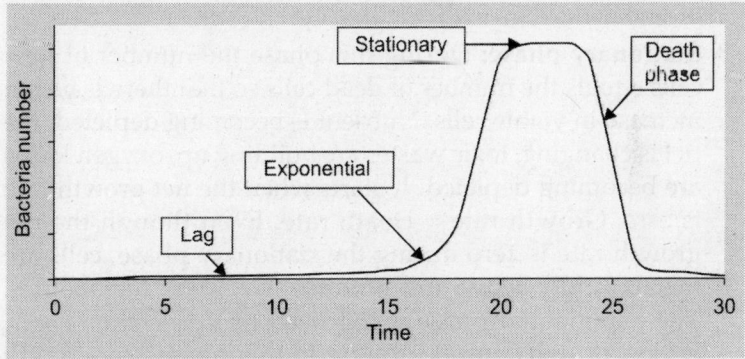

Fig. 9.6: Graph showing bacterial growth curve

Bacterial Growth Phases

1. **Lag phase:** Where the organisms are "getting used to the medium and physical conditions"—that is, they are inducing the necessary enzymes for growth. No increase in cell number Period of adaptation of cells to a new environment. No change in number, but an increase in mass. Multiple lag phases may sometimes be observed more than one carbon source *(Diauxic growth)*. Length of the lag phase—characteristics of microbial species and in part by the media conditions.

2. **Logarithmic (log) growth phase:** This is the phase where the generation time is measured. The more ideal the conditions, the faster the growth—up to the maximum growth rate for the species. Growth rate is higher. Increase in cell mass and cell number with time exponentially. This phase results in straight line. Hence, it is also known as *exponential phase*. Period of balanced growth, in which

all the components of a cell grow at the same rate. Composition of biomass remains constant. The exponential growth rate is the first order reaction. The rate of biomass is correlated with the specific *growth rate (μ)* and the biomass concentration or cell number, X. A measure of the rapidity of growth has dimension T – 1 dX/dt = μ.X .The exponential phase is followed by *deceleration phase,* period of unbalanced growth.

3. **Stationary phase:** During this phase the number of new cells equals the number of dead cells so that there is no net increase in viable cells. Nutrient is becoming depleted, the pH is changing, toxic wastes are building up, oxygen levels are becoming depleted. It starts when the net growth rate is *zero*: Growth rate = Death rate. Even though the net growth rate is zero during the stationary phase, cells are metabolically active and produce secondary metabolites. The exponential phase is followed by *deceleration phase,* period of unbalanced growth. In this phase, the growth decelerates due to either depletion of one or more essential nutrients or the accumulation of toxic byproducts of growth.

4. **Death phase:** Rate of cell death is faster than regeneration. Death may accelerate and become exponential. The specific growth rate is generally found to be a function of three parameters:

   1. The concentration of growth limiting substrate, S
   2. The maximum specific growth rate, μ_{max}
   3. A substrate-specific constant, Ks

Specific growth rate is independent of substrate concentration as long as excess substrate is present. It is represented by **Monod equation** given below.

$$\mu = \mu_{max}/Ks + S$$

The Monod equation is a mathematical model for the growth of micro-organisms. It is named for Jacques Monod who proposed using an equation of this form to relate microbial growth rates in an aqueous environment to the concentration of a limiting nutrient.

Nutrients Needed for Growth

Carbon Source

Organic compounds (heterotrophs)—glucose and other sugars, amino acids, sometimes complex preformed organic compounds (i.e. vitamins, **growth factors**), inorganic carbon (autotrophs) —carbon dioxide

Nitrogen

Nitrates and nitrites; elemental nitrogen if a nitrogen fixer. Amino acids and proteins (peptone, tryptone).

Oxygen and Water

Necessary for the growth and survival of micro-organisms.

pH

Most bacteria of medical importance prefer neutral pH: pH values in the range of 6–8. Exception: *Helicobacter pylori* which inhabits the stomach with a pH 1.

Temperature

Psychrophiles have a low temperature optimum (*Listeria monocytogenes* grows best at low temperatures, and cultures can be enriched by incubation at refrigerator temperature. **Mesophiles** have an optimum growth temperature around human body temperature. **Thermophiles** have a hot optimum growth temperature.

Cold temperatures are often used to slow microbial growth and thus preserve foods. Freezing tempertures do not kill microbes but preserve them in "suspended animation." Freeze-drying or **lyophilization** is often used to preserve microbial cultures.

KEY POINTS

- Microbiology is the study of all organisms that are invisible to the naked eye—that is, the study of micro-organisms, i.e viruses, bacteria, many algae and fungi, and protozoa.
- Micro-organisms are necessary for the production of bread, cheese, beer, antibiotics, vaccines, vitamins, enzymes.

- Classification of organisms: Living organism can be unicellular or multicellular.
- Unicellular organisms: The body of the organism is composed of single cell—prokaryotic in nature.
- Multicellular organisms: The body of the organism is composed of numerous cell—eukaryotic in nature.
- A species is a *class* of plants or animals whose members have the same *main* characteristics and are able to *breed* with each other.
- A strain is a low-level *taxonomic rank* used at the intra-specific level (within a *species*).
- Serotype is a sub-group of species, which are grouped according to their antigenic properties.
- Antigens are substances that are considered "foreign" to the host body.
- Taxonomy, in a broad sense—the science of classification-derived from the Greek *taxis* ("arrangement") and *nomos* ("law").
- Species: A collection of microbial strains that share many properties and differ significantly from other groups of strains.
- Strain: A population of organisms descended from a single organism or pure culture isolate.
- Morphology is the study of how things are put together. In morphology, the word part *morph-* means "form" and *-ology* "the study of".
- Vertical genetic transfer occurs when there is gene exchange from the parental generation to the offspring.
- Lateral/horizontal genetic transfer (LGT) is then a mechanism of gene exchange that happens independently of reproduction.
- Micro-organisms: Living organism (such as bacteria too small to be seen with naked eye but visible under a micro-scope).
- Antony van Leewenhoek (1632–1723) who invented the first microscope (50–300x) and was the first to accurately observe and describe micro-organisms.

- Methods of identification of micro-organism.
  1. Phenotypic method
  2. Phylogenetic method
  3. Other methods
     a. Numerical taxonomy
     b. DNA homology
     c. Ribosomal RNA homology
- Phenotypic method: The organisms can be classified on the basis of cell structure, cellular metabolism, or on differences in cell components.
- Phylogenetic analysis is to understand the past evolutionary path of organisms.
- Viruses: They are non-living particles with some chemical characteristics similar to those of living, but they do not have nucleus and cannot sustain independently and they require a host to carry out their biological activities.
- **Microscope** is an instrument that produces enlarged images of small objects, allowing the observer an exceedingly close view of minute structures.
- The eight types of microscopy are:
  1. Compound microscope
  2. Bright field microscopy
  3. Dark field microscopy
  4. Phase contrast microscopy
  5. Fluorescent microscopy
  6. Electron microscopy
  7. Transmission electron microscopy
  8. Scanning electron microscopy.
- Sterilization is making a substance free from all microorganisms both in vegetative and sparing states. Disinfection: Disinfection does not affect spore state organisms. The destruction or removal of all pathogenic organisms capable of giving rise to infection.
- Antiseptic: The term is used to indicate the prevention of infection, usually by inhibiting the growth of bacteria in wounds or tissues, e.g. dettol.
- Bactericidal: Those which able to kill bacteria.

- Bacteriostatic: Prevent multiplication of bacteria.
- Commonly used chemical for sterilization are alcohol, aldehyde, gases like 1. ethylene oxide, 2. beta propiolactone (BPL), 3. formaldehyde gas.
- Sterilization methods in laboratory are dry heat, flame sterilization and autoclaving.
- Sterilization is a process or killing all micro-organisms (including spores) on or in a material or object.
- Culture medium: The food material or substances required for growing micro-organisms *in vitro* (outside the body) is called culture medium.
- Composition of culture media
  1. Water
  2. Energy source
  3. Carbon source
  4. Nitrogen source
  5. Mineral salts
  6. Special growth factors
- Microbial growth kinetics: The relationship between the specific growth rate (μ) of a microbial population and the substrate concentration (s).
- **Bacterial growth curve:** When an organism is inoculated into a nutrient solution, four distinct growth phases are: 1. Lag phase, 2. logarithmic (Log) growth phase, 3. stationary phase, 4. death phase.
- Monod equation is $\mu = \mu_{max}/Ks + S$. It is mathematical model for the growth of micro-organisms.
- Nutrients needed for growth are carbon source, nitrogen, oxygen and water, pH, and temperature.

PRACTICE QUESTIONS

Very Short Answer Type Questions

1. What is microbiology?
2. Give two differences between unicellular and multicellular organisms.

3. Define: (a) Species, (b) strain, (c) serotype.
4. What is microscopy?
5. Give any two examples of commonly used chemicals for sterilization.

Short Answer Type Questions

1. Give the ecological importance of micro-organisms.
2. Give the characters of: (a) Prokaryotes, (b) eukaryotes.
3. Give the classification based on phylogenetic classification.
4. Write a note on compound microscope.
5. Give the importance of micro-organisms.

Long Answer Type Questions

1. What is microscopy? Explain about: (a) Bright field microscopy, (b) dark field microscopy, (c) phase contrast microscopy, (d) electron microscopy, (e) scanning electron microscopy and (f) fluorescent microscopy.
2. Write a note on sterilization and various techniques used.
3. Write a note on growth kinetics of micro-organisms.
4. Explain using a graph: (a) Lag phase, (b) log phase, (c) stationary phase and (d) death phase of micro-organisms.

Glossary

Abiotic factor	A nonliving component of an ecosystem.
Activation energy	The energy required to begin a chemical reaction.
Active transport	The movement of a substance across a cellular membrane from a region of lower concentration to a region of higher concentration using specific transport proteins and energy from ATP.
Adaptation	A characteristic that can improve an organism's ability to survive and reproduce in its environment.
Adenosine diphosphate (ADP)	A molecule that is formed during cellular energy release when an ATP molecule loses a phosphate group, and can be converted back to ATP by the addition of a phosphate group and energy.
Adenosine triphosphate (ATP)	A molecule that provides energy for many cellular activities. ATP releases energy when one of its high-energy bonds are broken by removing a phosphate group.
Aerobic respiration	A form of cellular respiration that requires oxygen to generate energy by converting glucose into CO_2 and H_2O and then using these molecules to produce ATP.
Allele	An alternative variation of a gene. Each gene has two alleles that interact to

produce a specific genotype and resulting phenotype.

Amino acid — A monomer or "building block" of a protein; there are 20 amino acids.

Anaerobic respiration — A form of cellular respiration that occurs in the absence of oxygen and produces ATP by breaking down glucose molecules (e.g. fermentation).

Anticodon — A sequence of three nucleotides in transfer RNA (tRNA). This sequence of nucleotides is complementary to the codon in the messenger RNA (mRNA) and corresponds with a specific amino acid during protein synthesis.

Artificial selection — A process in which humans breed organisms in order to increase or decrease the occurrence of specific genetic traits in offspring; also known as selective breeding.

Base-pairing — The principle that adenine should always chemically bond with thymine in DNA (or uracil in RNA) and cytosine should always bond with guanine during the formation of nucleic acids.

Biodiversity — A diverse group of different organisms in a given ecosystem or region at a specific time.

Biofuel — A fuel produced from biological materials (e.g. wood, ethanol, dried manure).

Biology — The branch of science that studies life.

Biome — A geographic area classified according to the dominant communities of organisms present who are in turn characterized by unique adaptations particular to that climate (e.g. desert, grassland, tropical rainforest). Biomes may be classified into land, marine, and freshwater biomes.

Biosphere	The part of Earth in which life exists and living organisms interact with their environment.
Biotic factor	A living component of an ecosystem.
Calvin cycle	A series of reactions occurring in the stroma of the chloroplast during photosynthesis, in which carbon dioxide is converted into high-energy compounds such as glucose and fructose.
Carbohydrate	A macromolecule in living organisms that is composed of carbon, hydrogen, and oxygen and functions to provide energy and structural materials for cells. Carbohydrates include sugars, starches, and cellulose.
Carbon cycle	The predictable pattern describing how carbon is used, recycled and reused in and throughout the earth.
Carnivore	A living organism that eats only animals.
Catalyst	A substance that accelerates the rate of a chemical reaction by decreasing the activation energy of the reaction without being changed by the reaction (e.g. enzyme).
Cell	The basic unit of all living things that is fundamental to the structure and function of the organism.
Cell cycle	The sequence of events in a cell life span including growth, duplication of genetic material, and division. The cell cycle consists of interphase, mitosis, and cytokinesis.
Cell membrane	The outer layer of a cell composed of phospholipids and proteins that separates the cell from its surroundings and controls the movement of substances in and out of

	the cell; this is also called the plasma membrane.
Cell wall	A rigid structure that provides support and surrounds the cell membrane in plant cells, bacteria, fungi, and some protists.
Cellular respiration	A complex set of chemical reactions in which chemical energy is transferred from organic molecules (e.g. glucose) and stored in the phosphate bonds of adenosine triphosphate (ATP) molecules for later use in energy-requiring activities of the cell.
Centriole	A short, cylindrical organelle composed of microtubules that are found in pairs in eukaryotic cells (except plants) and organizes the formation of a spindle during mitosis or meiosis in animal cells.
Centromere	A region that joins two sister chromatids and is the point where spindle fibers attach to pull the chromatids apart during mitosis and meiosis.
Charles Darwin	English naturalist who presented the scientific theory of evolution in his book *On the Origin of Species* (1859). Darwin presented scientific evidence of biological evolution and proposed natural selection as the mechanism for these changes over time.
Chemical energy	Energy that can either be released by a chemical reaction or absorbed by the forming of chemical bonds.
Chlorophyll	A green pigment within plant chloroplasts that capture solar energy so it can be converted into chemical energy.
Chloroplast	An organelle in plant cells and other eukaryotic photosynthetic organisms that is the site of photosynthesis.

Chromosome A structure of genetic material that is comprised of a linear strand of coiled DNA and associated proteins in the nucleus of eukaryotic cells, or as a circular strand of DNA in the cytoplasm of prokaryotic cells.

Codon A sequence of three nucleotides in messenger RNA (mRNA) which form a unit of genetic code that is interpreted by cells for the construction of proteins. The codon is complementary to the anticodon in the transfer RNA (tRNA).

Crossing-over A process that occurs during meiosis in which homologous chromosomes exchange segments of genetic material, resulting in chromosomes with new allele combinations contributing to overall genetic variability.

Cytokinesis The division of cytoplasm into two daughter cells during cell division, generally occurring during telophase.

Cytoplasm The contents of a cell that are within the plasma membrane.

Deoxyribonucleic acid (DNA) A double-stranded, helical nucleic acid molecule in the nucleus of eukaryotic cells and the cytoplasm of prokaryotic cells that encode the genetic information for living organisms.

Diffusion The natural movement of a substance from a region of higher concentration to a region of lower concentration; energy use is not required.

Diploid A cell that contains two sets of homologous chromosomes (2n), often one set is inherited from each parent.

DNA polymerase An enzyme that functions during DNA replication by joining individual nucleotides together to produce a new strand of DNA by using the original DNA strand as a template.

DNA replication The process in which a cell makes a duplicate copy of its DNA.

Dominant An allele or gene that is expressed in an organism's phenotype, even when paired with a recessive allele or gene.

Electron transport chain/system A stage of cellular respiration where a sequence of proteins use high-energy electrons to convert ADP into ATP.

Endocytosis The process where a cell takes in generally large substances from outside the cell through the formation of membrane-bound vesicles in the plasma membrane.

Endoplasmic reticulum (ER) An organelle in eukaryotic cells that is composed of membrane-enclosed sacs and produces and transports proteins and lipids. Rough ER has ribosomes on its surface for protein production. Smooth ER has no ribosomes, synthesizes steroids and lipids, and transports macromolecules.

Entropy The tendency of matter to progress toward increasingly disorganized states; a measure of the degree of disorder in a system.

Enzyme A protein that functions as a biological catalyst and accelerates the rate of a biochemical reaction by reducing the required activation energy of the reaction while remaining unchanged by the reaction.

Equilibrium The state of a chemical reaction where the concentrations of reactants and products have no net change over time.

Eukaryote A single-celled or multi-celled organism containing cells with a membrane-bound nucleus and usually other specialized membrane-bound organelles.

Evolution
Changes in the genetic composition of a population of organisms over multiple generations (microevolution) or the gradual development of new species of organisms from common ancestors over many years (macroevolution), as supported by scientific evidence.

Exocytosis
A process where a cell releases generally larger substances from the cytoplasm by discharging them as membrane-bound vesicles passing through the cell membrane.

Gamete
A specialized reproductive cell that contains half the number of chromosomes of a somatic cell (i.e. egg cell, sperm cell).

Gene
The essential unit of heredity that relates to a specific segment on a DNA strand. Genes control cell structure and function by coding for unique proteins.

Gene expression
The process where information contained in a gene is transcribed into mRNA and then translated into a protein to be expressed phenotypically.

Gene mutation
An alteration that changes a segment of DNA representing a gene.

Gene pool
The combined genetic information of every interbreeding organism in a particular population at any one time. In general, a large gene pool indicates high genetic diversity, and a small gene pool indicates low genetic diversity.

Genetic engineering
Techniques used for altering the genetic material of living organisms to produce particular desired functions and/or characteristics.

Genetic inheritance The passing of genetic information from parents to their offspring.

Genetic variability The tendency of genotypes in a population to be different from each other across the population.

Genetically modified organism (GMO) An organism whose genetic material has been altered by non-naturally occurring processes.

Genetics The scientific study of how genetic traits are passed on through successive generations of organisms.

Genotype The genetic makeup of an organism that determines the phenotypic expression of a particular trait or set of traits.

Genus A taxonomic grouping of related species, ranked below the classification level of family (plural—genera).

Geographic isolation Physical separation of population by a geographic barrier (e.g. mountain, canyon, body of water), likely preventing successful reproduction between the population and may result in speciation.

Glucose A specific carbohydrate molecule that functions as the main source of potential chemical energy in many organisms and is one of the primary products of photosynthesis in plants and other photosynthetic organisms.

Glycolysis The initial stage of cellular respiration where a molecule of glucose is broken in half, producing a net of two molecules of pyruvic acid (pyruvate) and two molecules of ATP.

Herbivore An organism whose primary diet consists only of plants.

Heterozygous	A genetic circumstance where an organism has two different alleles for a specific trait (e.g. Aa).
Homeostasis	The process where organisms maintain relatively stable internal environments despite changing environmental conditions.
Homologous chromosomes	A pair of chromosomes in a diploid cell that have corresponding DNA sequences with one coming from each parent; also called homologues.
Krebs cycle (citric acid cycle)	A stage of cellular respiration where pyruvic acid or pyruvate is broken down into carbon dioxide through a series of reactions to generate high-energy electrons for use in the electron transport chain to produce ATP.
Light-dependent reactions	The reactions in the chloroplast during the first stage of photosynthesis where light energy is captured by chlorophyll molecules and transferred to chemical energy to produce ATP and NADPH molecules.
Light-independent reaction	The second phase of photosynthesis where the Calvin cycle is carried out making sugars from the products of the light-dependent reaction.
Lipid	A macromolecule in organisms that is made of mostly carbon and hydrogen atoms and functions in long-term energy storage, insulation, and as a structural component in cell membranes. Lipids include fats, waxes, oils, and steroids.
Lysosome	A membrane-enclosed organelle in eukaryotic cells that contain digestive enzymes to break down food particles or eliminate waste products inside a cell (e.g. organelles, engulfed viruses, bacteria).

Macromolecule	A large molecule (polymer) composed of many smaller organic molecules called monomers. There are four types of biological macromolecules: Proteins, carbohydrates, lipids, and amino acids.
Meiosis	A two-stage process of cellular division that occurs in sexually reproducing organisms and results in four daughter cells, gametes, with half the number of chromosomes than the original parent cell.
Messenger RNA (mRNA)	A type of RNA molecule that is transcribed from DNA and carries an instructional template for the assembly of amino acids into proteins. In a eukaryotic cell, Messenger RNA leaves the nucleus and attaches to ribosomes in the cytoplasm for protein synthesis.
Metaphase	The second stage of mitosis and meiosis, during which chromosomes align along the equator of the cell.
Mitochondrion	A membrane-enclosed organelle in most eukaryotic cells that is the site of cellular respiration (plural—mitochondria).
Mitosis	A process where a eukaryotic cell divides to result in two somatic daughter cells, each containing the same number of chromosomes and genetic content as the original cell.
Monosaccharide	The monomer of a carbohydrate molecule, often known as a simple sugar (e.g. glucose, fructose, ribose).
Monohybrid cross	A model used to predict the inheritance pattern of a single differing trait in two individuals.
Monomer	A molecule that can chemically react with other like molecules to form a larger molecule called a polymer.

Mutation	A random change in the DNA nucleotide sequence of an organism. Mutations found in gametes can be inherited (e.g. chromosomal mutations, gene mutations) and mutations are often a source of genetic variation.
Nitrogenous base	An organic molecule that contains the element nitrogen. DNA contains the nitrogenous bases adenine, thymine, cytosine, and guanine while RNA contains the nitrogenous bases adenine, uracil, cytosine, and guanine.
Nucleic acid	An organic macromolecule that carries and stores genetic information. This macromolecule contains hydrogen, oxygen, nitrogen, carbon, and phosphorus, and the two kinds of nucleic acids are ribonucleic acid (RNA) and deoxyribonucleic acid (DNA).
Nucleolus	A structure that functions in ribosomal RNA (rRNA) synthesis and the formation of ribosomes; it is composed of proteins and nucleic acids and is found within the nucleus of a cell.
Nucleotide	The basic unit or monomer of a DNA or RNA molecule, consisting of a five-carbon sugar molecule, a phosphate group, and one of four nitrogenous bases (i.e. adenine, thymine/uracil, cytosine, guanine).
Nucleus	A membrane-enclosed organelle in eukaryotic cells that contain genetic information stored in DNA molecules and works to maintain the integrity of DNA and to control cellular activities by regulating gene expression.
Offspring	A new organism produced by one or more living organisms.

Omnivore   An organism whose primary diet consists of both plants and animals.

Organ   A group of tissues working together to perform a singular function or multiple functions, e.g. plant

Organic molecule   A molecule made up of large carbon-based structures that is found in or produced by living organisms (e.g. carbohydrates, lipids).

Organism   A single living cell or group of cells that make up one living thing, such as a plant or animal.

Osmosis   The movement of water molecules across a permeable membrane from a region of high water molecule concentration to a region of low water molecule concentration without requiring the use of energy.

Oxygen cycle   The predictable pattern describing how oxygen is used, recycled, and reused in and throughout the earth.

Passive transport   The act of substances moving into or out of a cell without the use of cellular energy.

pH scale   A system of measurement ranging from one to fourteen that indicates the relative concentration of hydrogen ions (H^+) in a solution. A pH of one indicates a strong acid while a pH of fourteen indicates a strong base, and a pH of seven is neutral.

Phenotype   The physical expression of a particular genetic trait, or genotype, which is influenced by an organism's genetic makeup and surrounding environmental pressures.

Phospholipid   A type of lipid that has a hydrophilic head and two hydrophobic tails and is primarily used as a structural component in cellular membranes.

Phospholipid bilayer
A double layer of phospholipids that provide structure for the cell membrane. The hydrophilic heads face the internal cytoplasm and external cell environment while the hydrophobic tails face inward toward each other.

Photosynthesis
A process involving a complex set of chemical reactions where plants and other organisms use sunlight energy to convert water and carbon dioxide into oxygen and high-energy carbohydrate molecules such as simple sugar

Polypeptide
A molecule produced when a series of amino acids are linked together by peptide bonds. Polypeptides are formed during the translation process of protein synthesis.

Polysaccharide
A complex carbohydrate composed of a chain of monosaccharides bonded together (e.g. cellulose, starch, glycogen).

Prokaryote
A single-celled organism that lacks a membrane-bound nucleus and membrane-bound organelles and has a nucleoid region in the cytoplasm containing a single, circular molecule of DNA.

Prophase
The first stage of mitosis and meiosis, during which chromatin condenses to form chromosomes, the nuclear envelope disappears, and the spindle begins to form.

Protein
A three-dimensional macromolecule in organisms that is composed of monomers called amino acids and contains carbon, hydrogen, oxygen, and nitrogen; perform many structural and regulatory functions in cells

Protein synthesis
The process in which proteins are produced, including the transcription of DNA to mRNA and the translation of mRNA to a polypeptide chain.

Punnett square	A diagram used to determine possible combinations of offspring alleles by crossing the alleles of parents with known genotypes. A Punnett square is used to predict the probability of offspring having certain allele combinations.
Recombinant DNA technology	The technology of producing altered DNA by cutting up DNA molecules from more than one organism into fragments and splicing the fragments together in a host organism.
Respiratory system	An organ system that brings oxygen into an organism, performs gas exchange, and then releases carbon dioxide back to the surrounding environment.
Ribonucleic acid (RNA)	A single-stranded nucleic acid molecule in the nucleus of eukaryotic cells and the cytoplasm of prokaryotic cells; consists of nucleotide monomers containing the sugar ribose, a phosphate group, and the nitrogenous bases adenine, uracil, cytosine and guanine. RNA functions as a messenger carrying instructions of DNA during protein synthesis.
Ribosomal RNA (rRNA)	A type of RNA molecule that is the main structural and functional component of ribosomes and the site of protein synthesis.
Ribosome	Composed of RNA and proteins that function at the site of protein synthesis in the cytoplasm of eukaryotic and prokaryotic cells.
Species	In classification of organisms, the lowest taxonomic grouping consisting of organisms that are capable of reproducing to produce fertile offspring.
Taxonomy	The branch of biology that focuses on classifying and naming organisms.

Telophase

The fourth stage of mitosis and meiosis, during which chromosome separation is completed, chromosomes uncoil, the spindle breaks down, and daughter nuclei form at the two poles of a cell. Cytokinesis usually begins during telophase.

Temperature

A measure of average kinetic energy of the particles in a sample of matter determining how hot or how cold that substance is. This measurement commonly uses the Celsius or Fahrenheit scale.

Tissue

A group of similar cells organized to perform one or more specific functions in a multicellular organism.

Trait

A specific characteristic in an organism that is expressed by genes and/or influenced by the surrounding environment.

Transcription

The process in which part of the nucleotide sequence of DNA is used as a template to synthesize a strand of messenger RNA (mRNA).

Transfer RNA (tRNA)

A type of RNA molecule that brings amino acids to the site of the ribosomes during protein synthesis.

Translation

The process in which the genetic information encoded in a strand of messenger RNA (mRNA) is decoded by a ribosome to produce a sequence of amino acids (called a polypeptide chain) for protein synthesis.

Vestigial structure

A structure in an organism that is functionless or incompletely developed. This is typically a structure more fully developed and functional in the organism's ancestors.

Water cycle

The predictable pattern describing how water is used, recycled, and reused in and throughout the earth.

X chromosome	One of the sex-determining chromosomes that is present in humans.
Y chromosome	One of the sex-determining chromosomes that is present in humans.
Zygote	The diploid cell formed after a sperm and egg unite.

Index